Technique and Interpretation

Autopsy of the Horse

ALSO BY JAMES R. ROONEY...

BIOMECHANICS OF LAMENESS IN HORSES
The Williams & Wilkins Company Baltimore, 1969

WITH WOLFGANG O. SACK AND ROBERT E. HABEL...

GUIDE TO THE DISSECTION OF THE HORSE
W. O. Sack, Ithaca, 1967

Autopsy

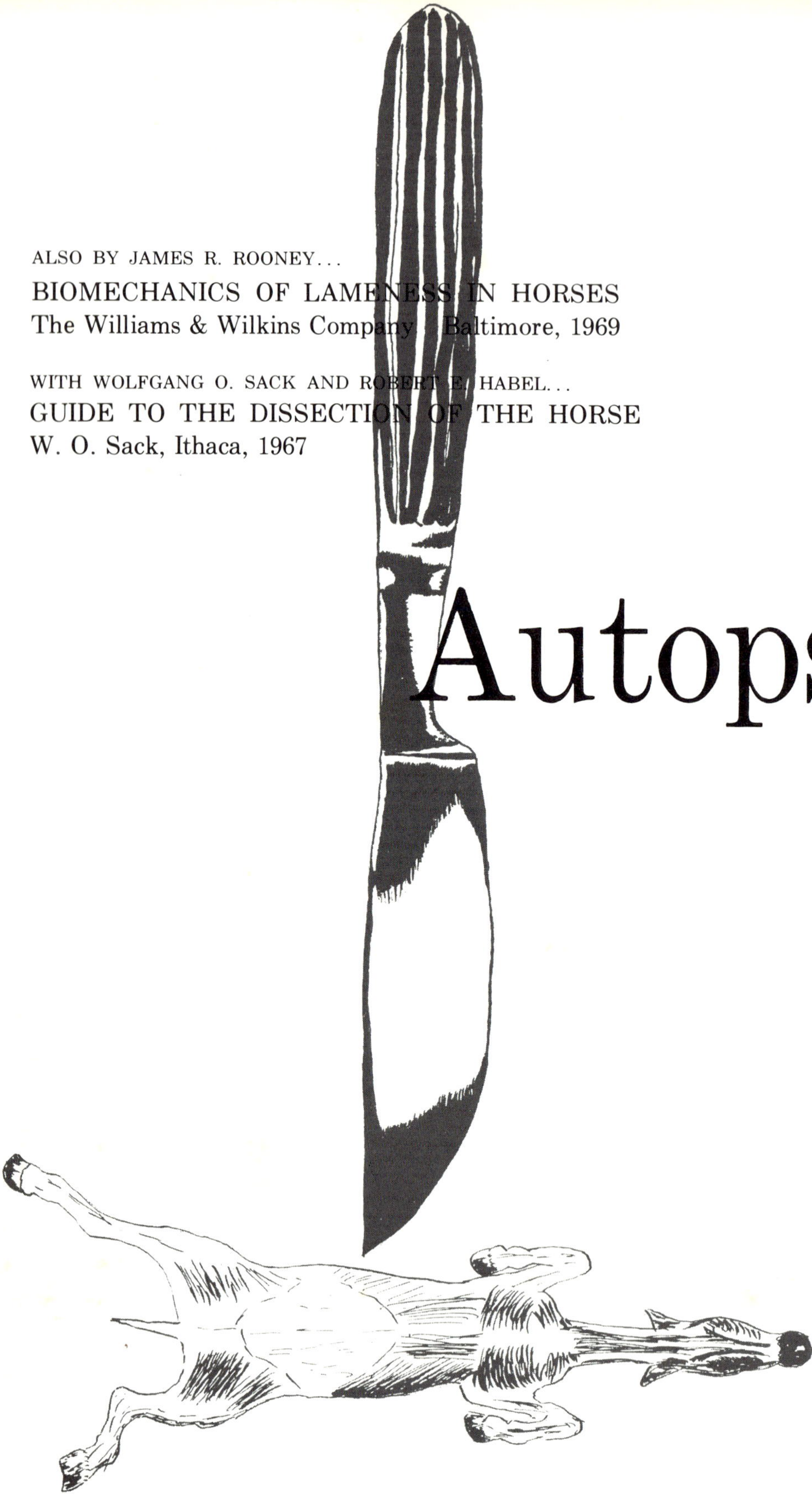

Technique and Interpretation

of the Horse

JAMES R. ROONEY, D.V.M.

Associate Professor of Pathology
School of Veterinary Medicine
University of Pennsylvania
Kennett Square, Pennsylvania

The Williams & Wilkins Co./Baltimore 1970

Made in the United States of America

Library of Congress Catalog Card Number 72-113631
SBN 683-07344-3

Composed and printed at the
Waverly Press, Inc.
Mt. Royal and Guilford Aves.
Baltimore, Md. 21202, U.S.A.

This book is dedicated
to My Parents,
with Love and Thanks.

Preface

This book is the work of a generalist, a pathologic anatomist with wide experience, some understanding and a great need to understand more. In the present day it is very difficult for any one man to comprehend all that should be comprehended in any area of human knowledge. Even though I have restricted this book—and myself—to the pathology of the horse, it is clear enough that all the facets of equine pathology cannot come within my ken.

The attempt, therefore, is not to present a compendium of equine pathology or solutions to the many unsolved problems of equine disease. This book is a record of my experience, what I think I know and what I think I want others to know.

Further, this book is a crusade. The autopsy technique described is based on the German system as learned by the author some years ago at the Royal Veterinary College, Stockholm, Sweden. That basic procedure has been modified and elaborated extensively, particularly for the locomotor system. While an autopsy can be carried out by a careful prosector, utilizing any technique, I feel strongly that the method presented lends itself to rapid, thorough, systematic work better than any other. There can be no disagreement unless and until this method has been given a fair test. I spent some years autopsying animals placed on the side and many more on the back; you must at least try the back before coming down on the side of the side.

Concerning the word autopsy: it has become fashionable to use necropsy for the animal and reserve autopsy for the human. There is no purpose in an involved semantic argument. Since the original Greek word means "viewing with one's own eyes," I believe the word autopsy to be quite appropriate and see no need for a pedantic change to necropsy—"viewing death." Those who disagree may substitute "nec" for "aut" where appropriate.

I am deeply indebted to the many veterinarians who have provided the many horses for my knife. Even more I am indebted to them for their clinical histories, accumulated experience and often incisive in-depth discussion of the relationships of clinical and autopsy findings.

I wish, particularly, to acknowledge the help, consultation and simple friendship of Dr. Lennart Krook, Dr. F. Michael Delaney, and Dr. Milton E. Prickett. Without them this book would have been neither conceived nor foaled.

Mrs. Marian Mochow, Miss Virginia Ransdell and Mrs. Grace Plate have suffered quietly through many slides and many rewritten words.

Mr. Melvin Jenkins, deceased, was for many years my strong right arm for every autopsy—days, nights and weekends. I shall miss him.

The publisher and, particularly, G. James Gallagher and George Gebhardt have been more than kind; they have been friends.

Introduction

This is a book about gross pathology, specifically the gross pathology of the horse. I intend to carry you through an autopsy procedure, the proper interpretation of what is observed during that procedure and last, and most important, help you develop an appreciation and understanding of what gross pathology is and what it means.

I write of the horse because I know more about that animal than any other. The reader should always bear in mind, however, that much of what will be said is of general significance, meaning, and import. Certain specific points refer only to the horse, but the overall philosophy, the methods of examining tissues and interpreting the size, shape, position, color and consistency (not to mention odor) is basic to all animals—two-legged or four-legged, hoofed or horned. No attempt will be made to discuss all the diseases of the horse; this is not so much a compendium or textbook of pathology as it is a working manual of technique and interpretation. Lead references will be provided from the voluminous literature on equine diseases.

There are several major themes which, I hope, will be discernible as the narrative unfolds. In order to be certain, however, I shall state them now and hope that you will find them apparent later.

It is my firm conviction that an autopsy is the rapid, systematic performance of an anatomical dissection. An autopsy is not conducted in order to expose lesions and facilitate their rapid passage from the steaming carcass to the stinking formaldehyde. Every autopsy should be so performed that the prosector sees all the relevant anatomical parts in proper structural and functional relationship to one another. Lesions should be seen in context and evaluated in context before culturing, fixation, etc. The autopsy should provide for the prosector a thorough review of the normal anatomical construction and appearance of the animal concerned.

A second and closely related point is completeness. It is not enough to find an abscess and stop, announcing to all and sundry that the postmortem is complete. As the clinician, seeing a down cow and administering calcium without examination of the udder or uterus, may well miss the most significant part of the sick animal, so the pathologist, by stopping at an obvious lesion, may miss a less obvious but more important or interesting lesion.

If the autopsy is performed as a complete anatomical dissection, the prosector will over a period of time automatically become proficient in the primary skill or characteristic of a pathologist: the ability to interpret. This characteristic cannot be taught; it can only be learned. The pathologist must know first when a given tissue or organ is normal. Normal is not a single thing, state or condition. Rather, it is the range of color, shape, size, and consistency which is normal for that particular thing in that particular species of animal. The synovial fossae in the humeroradial joint and tibiotarsal joint of the horse, for example, can vary widely and considerably in size and shape. In the young foal the fossae are not present. If the pathologist's sole experience with the humeroradial joint is the foal, he may well consider the normal fossae of the older animal as an osteoarthrosis. Such an error has appeared in the scientific literature.

An outstanding example is the spleen. I have frequently been asked, particularly by medical researchers, to define in quantitative terms the normal size and weight of the spleen in the Thoroughbred horse. After considerable experience it is my conviction that there is no such thing as a range or mean for these values in the horse. Each spleen must be considered in relation to the particular animal to which that spleen belonged. One must interpret the significance of the size and shape of the spleen in view of the conditions in the rest of the carcass. Numerical ranges and means are meaningless.

One cannot do one autopsy a month or one a year and consider himself a pathologist. Many spleens must be puzzled over, many tendons palpated, many tonsils sliced before the spectrum of normal becomes apparent.

A second feature of the pathologist's armamentarium must be the proper interpretation of agonal changes. I know of no area of greater confusion amongst students and part-time pathologists than this. Autopsy descriptions in the veterinary literature abound with descriptions of epicardial and endocardial hemorrhages, emphysema of the lungs and focal enteritis. As we shall see, most such changes occur as the animal is dying—during the terminal, agonal period. They are not unimportant changes, but their importance must not be exaggerated and misinterpreted in the search for etiology.

A third chapter of the pathologist's book of tricks must be the proper interpretation and differentiation of antemortem versus postmortem change. The significance is obvious, and most pathology training programs emphasize such differentiation.

Once the prosector has learned the normal, the agonal, and the rotten, the easy work is over. The hard part follows. He must look at all he has seen, consider his interpretation of the meaning of each individual change in each individual organ and tissue, and then correlate all the lesions, developing a reasonable, if not exact, interpretation: the natural history of the particular animal as far back as the lesions extend in time. It is immediately apparent that the prosector cannot simply view an organ as normal or abnormal; he must endeavor to determine the age of the changes present in that organ. Usually this is not the detective story type of determination: "This person died at 10:00 P.M. on Guy Fawkes' Day." Rather, one is more often concerned with the age of a lesion in relation to the age of another lesion in the same carcass. For example, is the exudate in the chest cavity of more recent origin than that in the peritoneal cavity? If so, we may consider that the peritonitis occurred first, followed by extension to the chest. Needless to say, one must search out the cause of the peritonitis; did it arise from the abscess in the liver or from infection introduced at the time of laparotomy?

Aging of lesions is often difficult and may be impossible. While the following remarks may be helpful, experience is the only real teacher. Rokitansky's principles apply directly: size, shape, position, color, and consistency. Larger lesions, if well organized, are generally older than smaller lesions. Total necrosis of the liver (Theiler's disease) is, however, an extensive lesion of short duration while small, focal, parasitic nodules may be of very long duration. Irregular shapes generally mean younger lesions, before invasion and growth in size have been limited by the defense mechanisms.

The position or location of a lesion is occasionally helpful. Lesions in critical areas of the brain and heart, for example, often are quickly lethal and therefore of short duration. Obviously the clinical history is vital.

The color and consistency of a lesion are probably the most useful criteria. The lighter and clearer the color, the younger the lesion, on average. Soft friable lesions are generally younger than firm tough lesions. When necrosis is present in an old lesion, however, the significance obviously changes. An old tumor with hard fibrous walls may have a young necrotic center. Calcification obviously implies age, but the horse calcifies lesions very rapidly and discretion is needed.

During the interpretation of a case the prosector is frequently confronted by the problem of related and unrelated lesions. It may be quite obvious that an arthrosis in the carpal joint is not related to volvulus of the small intestine. On the other hand, is the pleuritis related to the purulent endometritis or are they unrelated (but, nevertheless, both important!)? A horse has severe verminous thrombosis of the ileocecocolic artery and dies with acute streptococcal myocarditis. Did the thrombosis directly, indirectly, or not-at-all contribute to the death of the animal? We shall examine these matters as we go along.

Every autopsy has, I think, what might be called philosophical implications. Each pathologist, as each clinician, has his own way of doing and thinking and no amount of my verbiage will change that state of affairs. For what it might be worth, however, I should like to present my "philosophy." I do not believe it is the pathologist's task only to record lesions in clear, concise, descriptive language nor to use these descriptions to confound, confuse, and amaze the clinicians at clinicopathologic conferences. All too often the pathologist sees himself as the only man with the "answer" and makes perfectly obvious his disdain for the lowly brute who has so badly misinterpreted the clinical signs.

Even without an attitude of hauteur, however, the pathologist may be unwilling to meet his clinical colleague halfway: "These are the postmortem findings and this the pathologic anatomical diagnosis. Beyond these words I shall not pass."

I believe this is wrong. The failure of the clinician is truly and deeply the failure of the pathologist. The pathologist must be the teacher of the clinician. His is the opportunity to see the whole case, to review the clinical signs and explain those signs in terms of both pathologic anatomy and physiology. The pathologist's contribution must not be exclusively a well documented protocol, although that is basic. He must bring that protocol to life; he must perform that protocol like a play upon a stage, so that the clinician understands and calls for curtain call after curtain call. The clinician may even purchase a season ticket!

Often, I think, it is the pathologist's lack or narrowness of vision which is at fault. He must be willing to tread upon unsure ground, to attempt reasonable explanations and interpretations in the absence of solid fact. The clinician must interpret on a limited set of signs; surely the pathologist can do as much with even more signs—the clinician's findings plus his own.

An example may help to make the point. A yearling Thoroughbred was steadily losing weight over a period of weeks. According to the clinician there were no other significant clinical signs and the cause of the weight loss could not be determined. Eventually the animal was destroyed. At autopsy there was a marked malformation of cervical vertebrae three and four accompanied, microscopically, by demyelinization of the ventral two-thirds of the white matter of the spinal cord.

The clinician was irate on two counts. First, he could not believe the animal was ataxic—but had he really looked? The signs of ataxia may well be subtle and apparent only when the animal is turned in short, tight circles (perhaps this case made the point with this particular clinician, and he will recognize the next one). Secondly, he was disturbed that no lesion was found which could directly relate to the weight loss. I could not supply the lesion but, despite the absence of solid fact, felt justified in suggesting that severe pain, direct and/or referred from the cervical lesion, could have caused anorexia. Certainly this is uncommon in wobblers, but is it unreasonable for an individual case?

The clinician then supplied the missing links: the animal lost weight because he would not eat, and there was obvious reluctance to move the neck and head. Perhaps the horse could not reach the food because he was unwilling, because of pain, to lower his head to the ground!

The numerous special examinations which may be carried out to supplement the gross autopsy findings may play a significant role in the development of an exact interpretation of the natural history of the disease process. I think it is important to recognize, however, that these are *supplemental* examinations. In one of the examples given above the bacteriological findings are of immense importance. The cause of the myocarditis may never have been discovered unless the heart muscle was cultured. In order to answer the question posed, however, the thrombus would have to be cultured, also. If streptococci were present in the thrombus, one could reasonably interpret the case as myocarditis arising as a result of metastasis of infection from the thrombus to the heart muscle. The bacteriological findings, therefore, are only as important as the judgment of the prosector, at the time of autopsy, in selecting the appropriate culture sites. And, needless to say, that judgment is largely dependent upon a complete postmortem which included not only the obviously damaged heart but also the cranial mesenteric artery.

Similarly, histopathological examination is a higher power look, an extension of the naked eye examination in the postmortem room. There is, perhaps, nothing so worthless as detailed microscopic examination of a piece of tissue which was neither carefully examined nor described in the gross.

Virological studies, radiography and many other techniques may be employed as extensions and supplements to the gross examinations. They shall be considered in more detail later. At this point, I can only reemphasize that in the autopsy examination they are supplementary—they do not stand alone.

To conclude this chapter I should like to consider further, for a few moments, the relationship of the clinician and the pathologist. The pathologist is the handmaiden of the clinical sciences. It is his task to help the clinician improve his skills and understanding with every biopsy and every autopsy.

The pathologist serves the clinician directly by performing a thorough, complete autopsy on an individual case, constructing as reasonable a natural history of the disease process as possible and correlating his interpretation and findings with the interpretation and findings of the clinician. In order to carry out this function efficiently and well the pathologist must have the complete confidence, cooperation, and honesty of the clinician. Suspected clinical errors of judgment should not be hidden or glossed over. They may well out in any case, and, if they do not, the clinician and pathologist are both the losers because all aspects of the case have not been scrutinized before the final interpretation is made.

Under ideal circumstances the clinician may well call in the pathologist for discussion of the case before death. Such consultation not only enlivens and makes more meaningful the autopsy specimen but provides the opportunity for meaningful interchange of ideas between the clinician and pathologist.

Contents

ONE

Preparation and Initial Dissection

Preparation

Although the equipment and facilities for performing the autopsy vary from place to place, certain basic fundamentals must be available and certain basic procedures followed.

For the horse and other large animals the autopsy table shown in Figure 1 has been designed for the autopsy procedure described herein. In the absence of such a table, an arrangement which will allow the animal to be placed and held on its back on the ground or floor is satisfactory, although less convenient. The prosector and an assistant roll the animal up on its back, and the prosector cuts down all four limbs, as described below, while the assistant maintains the animal in dorsal recumbency. Once the limbs have been laid down further external support is unnecessary. If the horse is lean and high-withered or if the neck muscles are in rigor, the carcass may lean to one side or the other. It is desirable to have the carcass lean slightly to the animal's right because the viscera will be removed on that side. The head and neck may be used as a rudder to determine the position of the carcass. When the head is pulled around to the animal's left the carcass leans to the right; when it is pulled around to the right the carcass leans to the left. When the head is straightened out the carcass will be upright.

Often, during discussions and demonstrations of this autopsy procedure, practitioners complain that they cannot do field autopsies because of the policies of local rendering companies. It is a shame to hamper veterinary medicine on such grounds, and perhaps a compromise could be effected.

Usually the practitioner goes to the rendering plant and watches as the carcass is torn to pieces, in the hope of seeing something which he can relay to his client. I suggest that the practitioners in an area discuss with the renderer the possibility of providing a small space at the plant for the proper performance of the autopsy. The practitioners could have a table constructed. The renderer could skin the carcass to his own satisfaction and place it on the table. Upon completion of the autopsy the renderer would have the eviscerated carcass and the viscera, and part of his work will have been done for him and in his own plant. This plan of course requires the cooperation of the practitioners in an area—perhaps a more difficult problem than that of obtaining the cooperation of the renderer.

Ample water and protective clothing must be provided. I feel that it is essential

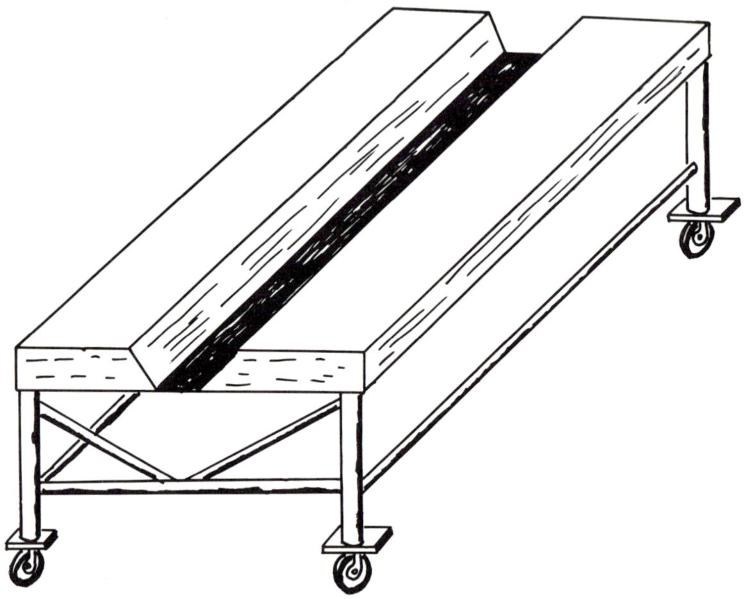

FIG. 1. Autopsy table. Tubular or angle frame. Rust-resistant top. Dimensions (approximate): height, 29 inches; width, 3 feet; length, 7 feet. Groove, 6 inches wide.

for the prosector to divest himself completely of his regular clothing and wear only coveralls and knee-high boots. If even the undergarments are not taken off, there is a tendency to back away from the necessarily messy carcass in order to protect oneself. Large animal autopsies cannot be done neatly if they are to be done thoroughly! A plastic or rubber apron which laps over the boots provides full length protection. When an autopsy is carried out on the ground, however, the apron only gets in the way and is best discarded. Concerning gloves, I plead heresy. I have never been able to see the point of gloves extending to my wrist or forearm when, as simple fact, blood and gore will extend at least to my elbow. One may say that gloves protect against cuts, but any knife worth using for an autopsy will cut a glove and hand as quickly as the bare hand. Indeed, because of the increased sensitivity of touch without gloves I believe there is less tendency to cut oneself. Rather than wearing gloves, I prefer to rinse my hands and arms frequently with clean water. The arms and hands should be wet at all times, allowing no blood or other fluids to dry on the skin. Such frequent rinsing and washing may seem time-consuming. However, one can while rinsing look at the carcass and think about what he has seen, what the interpretation of the case is up to that moment, and catch his breath. The time is not wasted.

A great variety of instruments may be employed in performing an autopsy, often with no other justification than that the prosector is pretending he is doing surgery. In fact, the only instruments required for the routine postmortem are an excellent steel, knife, Mayo (blunt point) dissecting scissors, rat-tooth long-handled forceps, and a good butcher saw. I cannot emphasize too strongly the quality and condition of the knife. It should be an expensive boning knife used exclusively for autopsies. After every use it should be carefully sharpened on a hand or motorized stone, dried, oiled carefully, and kept in a protective sheath. Once the blade thins noticeably from repeated sharpening the knife should be retired to other uses and a replacement secured. Many autopsies are not done simply because the prosector was sufficiently discouraged on his first attempts by a dull, miserable blade.

During the course of the autopsy the knife should be steeled frequently on a smooth or lightly ribbed steel. There is nothing more indicative of inexperience than manual awkwardness in steeling a knife. The veterinarian will practice knot-tying, graceful stomach-tubing, dextrous nerve blocking, and elegant firing, and the admiring client will say, "Doc sure is slick." That same veterinarian, however, will steel a knife as if the steel were red hot or were repelling the knife magnetically. Since some part of medicine still remains art and showmanship, I strongly urge some practice with the knife and steel. One cannot always count on the layman to run for air when the carcass is opened. As with hand rinsing, steeling is an excellent opportunity to catch one's breath, review what has been done, and consider what may be coming next. I believe the clinicians call this "syringe-filling," and I wholeheartedly subscribe to the practice.

Clinical history, including management conditions, nutrition, weather, etc., and the clinical pathology findings should be carefully reviewed before the autopsy begins. However, such information is not always available or is incomplete. Should the pathologist refuse to begin before such history is made available? I do not feel that the answer is as simple as may be at first assumed. Without a history certain important examinations may not be done, as in the case of spinal cord lesions when the cord is not routinely examined (and it never is) or the lesion is microscopic. Also, the prosector may be unnecessarily exposed to such diseases as rabies or encephalomyelitis. On the other hand, the historyless autopsy provides a fine intellectual challenge for the prosector. Can he unravel the natural history of disease in the animal by working with morphology alone? I believe that he can in many cases, and that the attempt is worth making. Age, sex, external examination, and the spectrum of lesions (or lack of lesions) provide the clues for what can be, if properly viewed, a challenging intellectual game. After all, why is the prosector a pathologist at all if not to respond mightily to such challenges? Understand that I am not advocating that autopsies be done routinely without clinical history, but neither am I advocating that they should never be done.

Dissection

Note that throughout this book *left, right, dorsal, ventral, cranial,* and *caudal* refer to the carcass itself, the animal's left, right, dorsal part or surface.

The animal is placed in dorsal recumbency either on the table with the aid of an electrical or mechanical hoist or on the ground. In the latter case the prosector and an assistant roll the animal up on the back and the assistant steadies it in this position. The entire surface of the body, all orifices, and the eyes should be examined.

Cut down both rearlegs by incising the skin, severing the medial muscles of the thigh, opening the hip joint, and transecting the round and accessory ligaments. The foreleg opposite the assistant is laid down by incising the skin and severing the pectoral muscles, vessels, and nerves, holding the knife close to the thoracic wall. The remaining foreleg is laid down, and the carcass is oriented by the head and neck "rudder" as described earlier.

The inexperienced prosector might do well to examine the vessels and nerves in the axillary space before laying the foreleg down completely. Incise the skin and pectoral muscles, and blunt and sharp dissect the major arteries and nerves. Anatomical review and practice of this type will eventually bear fruit, as with a case of radial paralysis, for example.

If the animal is on the table, the rearlegs should be cut down as described, but the hip joint is not opened and the ligaments are left intact. The rearlegs remain cocked up in the air which facilitates opening the pelvis.

Reflect the skin from the ventral surfaces of the head, neck, trunk, and medial surfaces of the limbs down to the coronary band. Do not skin the mammary glands, and leave a rim of skin around the anus and vulva. The prepuce, scrotum, and anus are not skinned.

In the female, dissect the udder free from the ventral body wall, working from the cranial edge and drawing the udder caudad, being careful to include the mammary (superficial inguinal) lymph nodes with the udder.

In the male, incise the scrotal skin and blunt dissect the tunica vaginalis parietalis from the skin. Free the tunica to the external inguinal ring with the ductus, etc., included. Open the tunica to determine the precise position of the testis.

Dissect the penis and sheath free from the ventral body wall caudad to the ischial arch. Carefully pulling the penis caudad, transect the crura of the penis as the penis curves

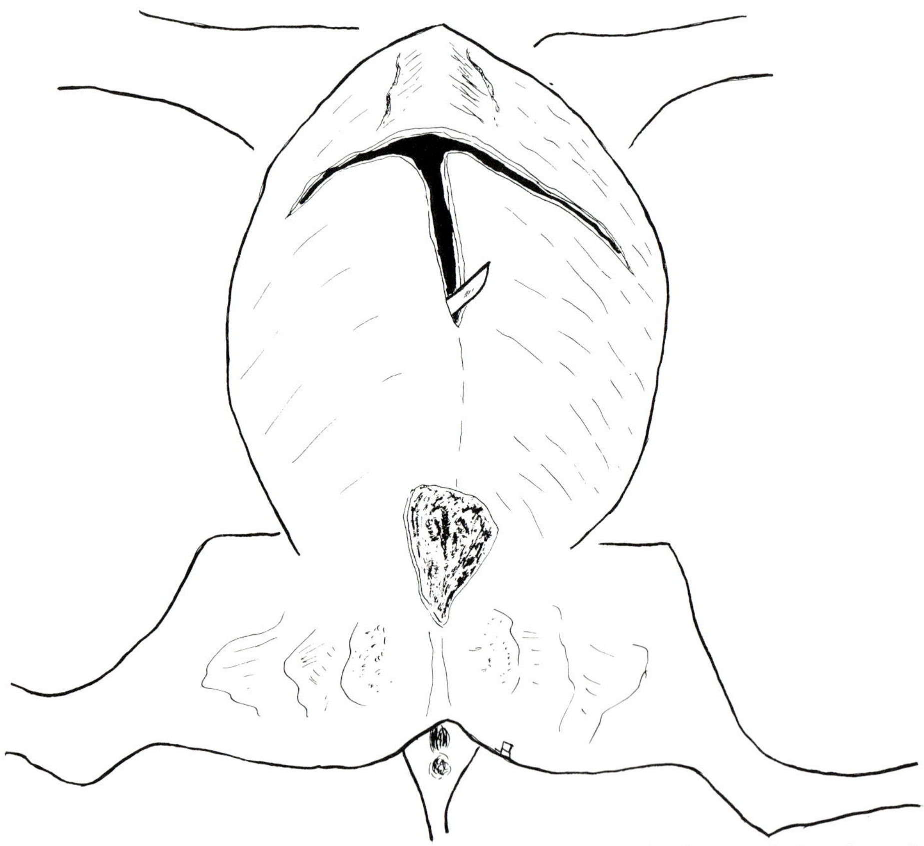

FIG. 2. Carcass in dorsal recumbency and skinned. The initial incision has been made into the peritoneal cavity. The incision is being carried along the ventral midline with the knife point out to avoid cutting the viscera. The mammary gland is shown *in situ* but would be removed before the peritoneal cavity is opened.

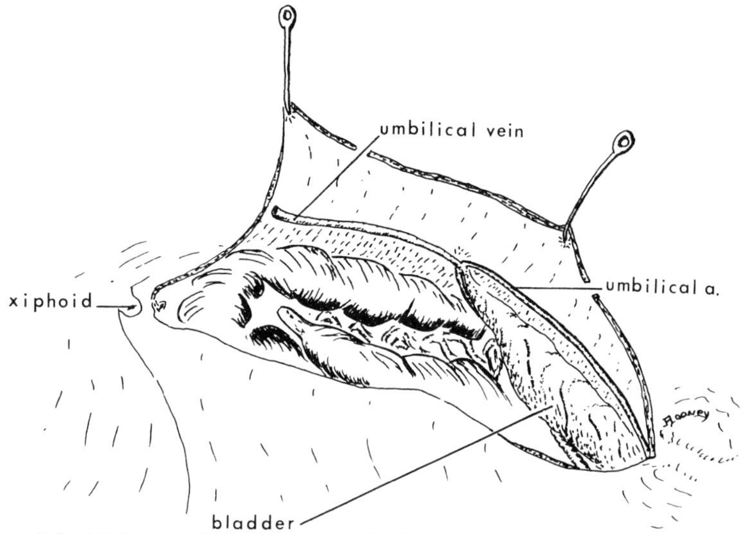

FIG. 3. Relationships of the bladder, umbilical artery, and vein in the foal before the bladder has separated from the umbilicus. The incision from xiphoid to pubis is placed just off the midline on either side in order to keep the bladder-umbilicus relationship intact. Only one incision is shown.

around close to the ischial arch. The dissection should be done carefully as the urethra is easily cut at this time. The same procedure is followed for the gelding with the obvious omissions.

The viscera table is drawn up on the animal's right. With the prosector standing on the animal's left, the peritoneal cavity is opened by an incision 5 cm. caudal to the xiphoid cartilage (Fig. 2).

In the fresh carcass, before gaseous distension of the large intestine becomes marked, the abdominal wall is tightly concave. The incision should be made down to the layer of retroperitoneal fat. Break through this fat and the immediately subjacent peritoneum with the fingers. The pressure within the abdomen is lower than the ambient pressure, and air will rush in, ballooning and loosening the abdominal wall.

When postmortem gaseous distension is marked, a similar procedure is followed. The distended cecum or colon will bulge outward, however, interfering with the subsequent dissection. Release the gas by a small knife puncture or punctures. It is better to release the gas knowingly and under control than have it burst forth from an inadvertently incised or ruptured gut.

Carry the incision caudad on the midline to the pubis, holding the knife point out to avoid cutting the viscera (Fig. 2). In the young foal carry the incision around the umbilicus on either side. The umbilicus-urachus-urinary bladder relationship must be maintained (Fig. 3).

Continue the incision laterally along the cranial border of the pubis on both sides. In the male incise the flank to and into the inguinal canal, freeing the ductus, vessels and testis (see Fig. 21, Chapter 2).

Reflect the left lateral abdominal wall by continuing the incision from the cranial end of the midline incision parallel and about 5 cm. from the curve of the last rib. This incision should not be carried so far that the viscera spill out on the left side.

The prosector should now move to the animal's right side and reflect the right lateral abdominal wall. Carefully observe the abdominal contents (Fig. 4) noting displacements, discoloration, etc. Allow and assist the cecum and dorsal and ventral colon to run out on the right side onto the viscera table or ground. Adjust the colon and cecum so that they are not twisted and the neurovascular complexes are uppermost. If using the table the prosector

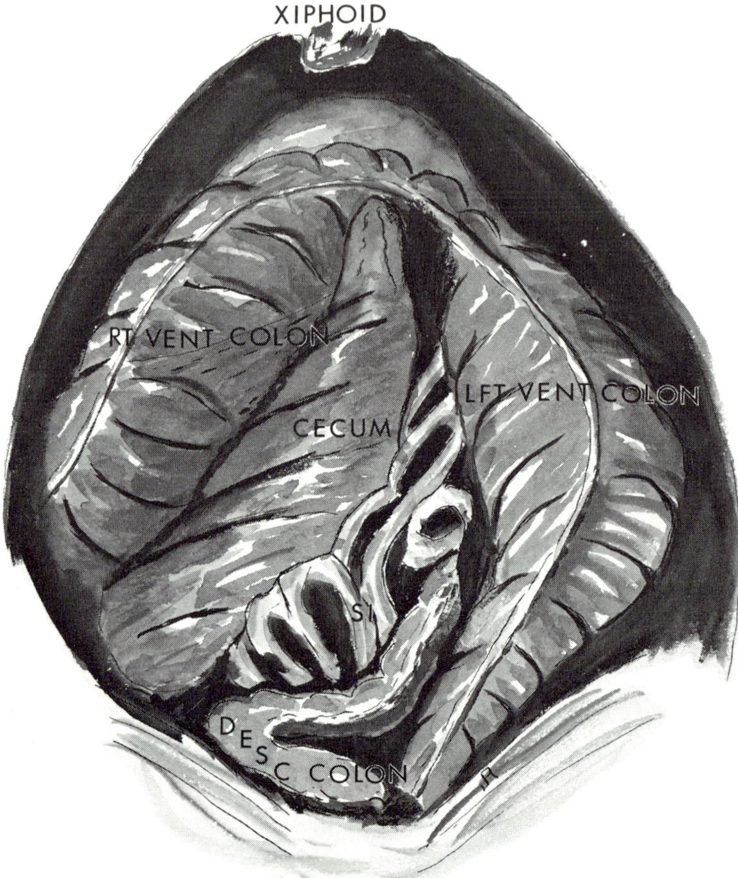

FIG. 4. Normal position of the abdominal viscera after the initial incisions have been made and the flanks laid down. The descending colon and small intestine may or may not be visible.

should (after properly adjusting the apron) wedge himself between the viscera table, flank of the animal, and the rearleg.

Interpretation

Skin

Rigor mortis develops in the muscles as follows: head, neck, back, foreleg, rearleg; it disappears in the same order. The timing of the onset of rigor varies enormously with body size, environmental temperature, fat, cause of death, etc.

The several body orifices should be examined for bleeding and ulceration. Postmortem prolapse of the rectum as a result of gaseous distension of the abdominal viscera is not uncommon. Except in the immediate postmortem period the mucosae are singularly uninformative. Although the mucosae are useful clinical indicators of the condition of the circulating blood, the blood quickly drains away and pools after death, and useful postmortem observations are difficult to obtain or interpret.

The haircoat should be carefully examined. With lightning stroke about 50% of the cases will have burned tracks in the hair from the area of the withers to or near the coronary band. These tracts, often very narrow and almost imperceptible, show as singeing of the hair with curling and frizzing.

Chronic disease processes such as malignancies, severe parasitic infestations, and chronic peritonitis may be accompanied by a dry, scurfy haircoat, patchy alopecia, and occasionally, intense pruritus. The elevated ulcerative lesions of habronemiasis (summer sores) preferentially involve the penis, sheath, legs, and skin of the ventral surface of the body. Areas of vitiligo along the ventral midline and around the eyes are usually caused by *Onchocerca* microfilaria.

The length of the haircoat should be noted with reference to the time of the year. The winter haircoat may be retained beyond the normal time in debilitated or chronically ill animals. Large adenomas of the intermediate lobe of the pituitary gland, pressing against the hypothalamus, may be associated with retention of the winter haircoat and excessively long haircoat.

Firing scars, scurf caused by blisters, and the like should be carefully noted both before and during removal of the skin. The lack of subcutaneous and/or deeper reaction to these superficial treatments will impress even the novice prosector.

Scars in the usual neurectomy areas (particularly metacarpus and digit) and scar tissue in the subcutaneous areas should be noted. Careful dissection of the relevant nerve trunks is required because of the medico-legal implications.

Lymphangitis, particularly of the rearlegs, is not common but is serious. *Sporotrichum schenckii* (48) is a known cause of this condition in North America, whereas *Histoplasma farciminosum* (39) and glanders (farcy) are not seen in North America. The cause of most cases of lymphangitis in North America is unclear. Streptococcus or *Corynebacterium ovis* are occasionally isolated, but their precise role—initiator or opportunist—is not clear.

Acute lymphangitis is characterized clinically by pain, heat, swelling, and, at autopsy, by extensive yellowish subcutaneous edema with pronounced distension of individual lymphatic channels with pus (Fig. 5). Chronic cases are characterized by massive subcutaneous fibrosis with scattered purulent foci (see below).

There are numerous skin conditions in horses, some well defined (ringworm, phycomycosis) (10, 11, 37) and others poorly defined. Skin changes should be saved for parasitological, mycological, and histological study, even though they have no relationship to the cause of death.

Two purposes are served by skinning the animal as extensively as has been prescribed. First, it is dangerous to attempt to open joints, the abdomen, or any deeper structure with the skin in place. The loose subcutaneous tissue allows the skin to slide about freely and, particularly during rapid work, the knife easily slips on the hair and sliding skin. Second, large areas of subcutaneous tissue are available for examination.

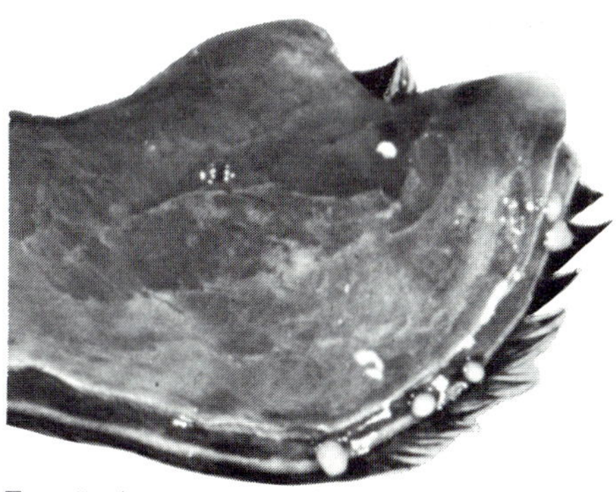

FIG. 5. Acute sporotrichosis. Subcutaneous lymphatics are distended with pus which can be seen oozing out from the cut edge.

Subcutaneous Tissue

The normal appearance of the subcutaneous tissues cannot be readily described but once it is appreciated the abnormal variations are easily recognized and of considerable assistance in the overall interpretation of the case.

Dehydration. The subcutaneous tissues are dry, tight, and crackling and the skin is removed with difficulty. Normally, small air bubbles are trapped in the loose connective tissue as the skin is pulled away. These should not be mistaken for the massive (and rare) air masses of subcutaneous emphysema. Such emphysema may occur following puncture wounds, particularly in the axillary area, and involve almost the entire surface of the body. Occasional cases of subcutaneous emphysema have been seen with no evidence of puncture wound or other cause. In any event, wound or no wound, recovery is usually uneventful, and there is rarely an occasion to autopsy such animals.

Asphyxial and Postmortem Changes. The subcutaneous tissues are muddy and a dull reddish-black. The vessels appear as a distinct, dense spider web network containing dark, tarry, nonclotting blood. In young foals this pattern is accompanied by a marked yellow tinge, in contrast to the dull, muddy appearance in the older animal.

The asphyxial pattern may be difficult to appreciate if the autopsy has been delayed. Postmortem decomposition produces the same discoloration and it may be impossible in some cases to differentiate the agonal, asphyxial pattern from postmortem decomposition.

The hyperemic vessels and discoloration may be more pronounced on one side than the other as a result of postmortem hypostasis. Significant hypostasis is not commonly seen unless asphyxial changes develop during the agonal period. One may tentatively, then, differentiate postmortem from asphyxial discoloration (in a delayed autopsy) by the absence or presence, respectively, of significant hypostasis.

It appears that the asphyxial pattern is primarily an agonal event, occurring during the last hour or half-hour of life when there is a toxic or septicemic process such as pleuritis, peritonitis, twisted intestine, or salmonellosis. If, for example, two horses develop a volvulus of the small intestine at the same time and one is destroyed one-half to one hour before the natural death of the second, the first animal may show only slight subcutaneous asphyxial changes as compared to the marked changes in the animal allowed to go through the agonal period.

When the skin is reflected from the cervical region, particular attention should be directed to the jugular veins for evidence of venipuncture and firm distension (thrombosis). Severe asphyxial hemorrhages are common in this area, however, and may mask bleeding from the jugular vein.

Icterus, Anemia. Very pale, lemon-yellow subcutaneous tissues signify severe anemia as a result of idiopathic anemia, equine infectious anemia, piroplasmosis, hemolytic icterus of foals, or hemorrhage. In the latter case, the hemorrhage may not be apparent externally, as in postparturient "bleeder" mares, for example.

Anemia is usually present in piroplasmosis (58) and is often present in animals dying of equine infectious anemia, but may not be present if the animal is destroyed. The anemic appearance of tissues may be obscured by asphyxial changes if the animal goes through the agonal period.

Icterus is exceedingly difficult to detect in the live horse or at postmortem. The normal, yellowish color of the mucosae, tunica flava abdominis, and intimal lining of arteries obscures all but the most obvious icteric discoloration. Icterus is clearly apparent only in the presence of profound anemia as a faint greenish-yellow tinge of the mucosae and, at autopsy, of the intimal lining of large vessels.

Edema. Pleuritis and cardiac disease routinely cause edema, particularly prominent along the ventral midline, which may extend into the rearlegs. Hemolytic diseases and anemias such as equine infectious anemia, on the other hand, cause a more diffuse edema involving all four legs as well as the tissues along the ventral midline.

Clear, subcutaneous edema of the prepuce, rearlegs, and less commonly the forelegs occurs often in heavily exercised horses "stood up" for long periods in a box or stall (stocking up). It readily disappears with exercise. Acute lymphangitis causes edema of the rearlegs, but the process is painful, there are overlying erosions of the skin, and the edema fluid is yellowish and/or tinged with red. Chronic lymphangitis is characterized by gradual conversion of the edema to hard, subcutaneous fibrosis.

Focal areas of yellowish (inflammatory) edema wherever located suggest the need for a diligent search for cause (wound, underlying fracture, etc.).

Anorexia, of whatever cause, eventually leads to inanition and cachexia. The normal fat deposits disappear (are mobilized for energy and not replaced) and are replaced by grayish, gelatinous edema fluid.

Bruising. Bruising, particularly near joints, suggests that the animal has been down and thrashing. If the subcutaneous hemorrhage is dark and dry and there are ulcerations of the overlying skin, the animal has been recumbent for some time, and the significance is not the same as that of the bright, fresh bleeding of the acute colic case, for example.

Localized subcutaneous bruising (edema and hemorrhage) may be seen, particularly in foals, with no evidence of damage to the overlying skin. Such bruises are generally on the thoracic wall and careful palpation may reveal underlying fractured ribs. It is singular that the blow of a horse's hoof may bruise the subcutaneous tissues and fracture ribs or rupture the liver or spleen without leaving a trace of damage to the skin or hair at the site of impact. Indeed, in some cases the spleen or liver may be ruptured with no evidence of superficial or subcutaneous damage; only a prior observation of the actual blow provides knowledge of the cause.

Muscular Changes. One may gain a general overview of the skeletal muscles after the skin has been removed. The medial thigh, pectoral, medial shoulder, and external intercostal muscles, among others, are immediately available for examination. Whitish discoloration of the pectoral muscles is not uncommon in animals that have been recumbent, usually involving one side more than the other. Hemorrhage in the shoulder or thigh muscles is not uncommon in horses that have been recently restrained for surgery. General Zenker's degeneration of muscle has been frequently described as a gross autopsy finding. In fact the fishflesh, slightly cooked appearance or grayish coloration of the skeletal muscle is most commonly postmortem degeneration (cloudy swelling).

If focal or well defined areas of whitish or hemorrhagic discoloration are seen, true degenerative changes, such as in azoturia or myolysis, may be present, and microscopic examination is indicated. If virtually all the skeletal muscle is pale, however, postmortem change is the most likely cause. "White muscle disease" has been seen in horses (24).

Other Changes

Not everything that can be found or deduced from examination of the subcutaneous tissues has been discussed. The intention (I hope apparent) is to show that there is much to learn as soon as the skin has been removed.

The mammary gland of the mare is singularly free of significant lesions. I have seen only a few cases of severe, chronic, fibrosing mastitis and two cases of mammary gland adenocarcinoma at autopsy. The dark, greasy material between the two halves of the udder is sebaceous secretion of the same nature as that seen in the sheath of horses (smegma).

Fluid in the cavity of the tunica vaginalis immediately suggests peritonitis. Looping of the small intestine in the cavity may be either an antemortem or postmortem event. In the former case (inguinal hernia), the loop will be distended, intensely red to black-red and adhered to the tunica vaginalis by strands and mats of fibrin. In the latter case, usually seen with advanced postmortem decomposition and distension, the loop will be pale and will not distend the tunica vaginalis parietalis significantly.

One should note carefully whether both testes are in the scrotum, at the external ring, or within the abdominal cavity (cryptorchid). In young foals the testes are normally in the scrotum or at the external ring. The large gubernaculum testis may appear to be a testicle in the scrotum when in fact the testis is still in the inguinal ring.

Lesions of the penis and sheath are apparently rare. Squamous cell carcinoma

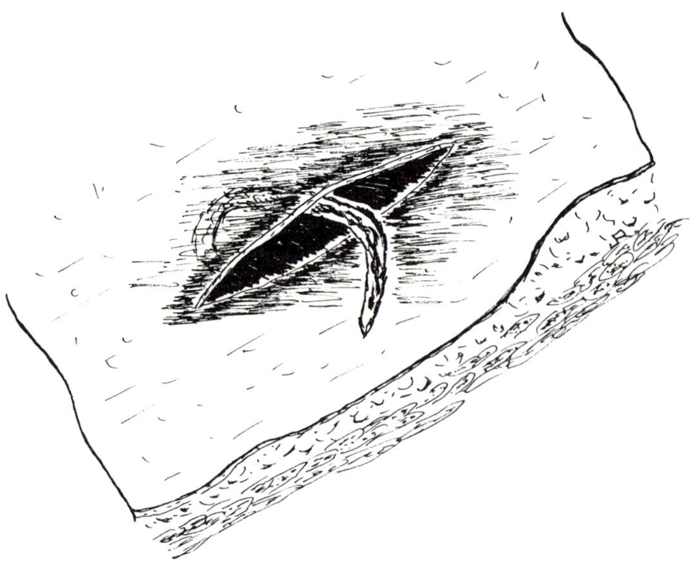

FIG. 6. *Strongylus edentatus* lesion. The larvae lie in the retroperitoneal tissue and can be recovered by incising the peritoneum and exerting gentle pressure.

of the prepuce, once frequently mentioned, is much less common in the modern, light horse era. The genital tract is discussed in greater detail below.

After the abdominal cavity has been opened, the prosector should stand directly to the rear of the animal to gain a thorough overview. The positions and condition of the cecum, ventral colon, descending colon and small intestine should be noted. Many forms of intestinal malposition are quite obvious at this stage. A distended large intestine, fluid-filled and with a bluish, cyanotic serosal surface, immediately suggests severe stasis of the large intestine (rotation, exhaustion shock, salmonellosis, infarction).

The spleen, liver, stomach, greater omentum, and diaphragm should be noted. The peritoneal surfaces of both flanks should be examined for the characteristic yellowish, edematous, hemorrhagic splotches caused by the larvae of *Strongylus edentatus* (Fig. 6). The larvae may be recovered by incising the peritoneum over the splotches. As a rule, with mild or moderate infestations the larvae are present only in the retroperitoneal tissues of the right flank. If they are present in the left flank as well, one may reasonably assume a severe infestation. I have never seen larvae in the left flank alone. It has been suggested that the larvae cause peritonitis, but I have not observed this relationship. Long, slender white worms may be found free in the peritoneal cavity (on the serosal surface of a viscus). These are *Setaria equina* adults, of no known pathological significance (46).

Old mares in particular, even though subsisting on grass and hay only, can become obese. The fat is deposited primarily in retroperitoneal tissues rather than in the subcutaneous tissues. External examination may not accurately indicate the true degree of obesity in a given animal. The subcutaneous tissues of older animals are usually much yellower in color than those of younger animals.

TWO

Evisceration of the Abdomen

Dissection

Removal of the Small Intestines

Standing on the animal's right, displace the descending colon out of the abdomen on the left side and draw the small intestines out on the right side. There is normally a small quantity (about 100 ml.) of clear yellow peritoneal fluid. Changes in color or amount should be noted.

With the small intestine displaced to the right, identify the duodenocolic ligament, between the ascending duodenum and the transverse colon, and break it down by blunt dissection with the fingers (the knife is of course sheathed in muscle). The duodenocolic ligament is the anatomical demarcation between the jejunum and the distal end of the ascending duodenum. Bluntly dissect the ascending duodenum to the caudal flexure (the anatomical junction with the descending duodenum). Pull on the duodenum until movement is apparent at the duodenopyloric junction and transect the duodenum. (Routinely, it is not necessary to ligate the gut before transection. If a viscus is markedly distended with fluid, ligatures may be placed at the prosector's discretion.) With this technique the duodenum will always be transected at or near the caudal flexure, which may be of importance when the intestine is examined later and one wishes to locate a lesion precisely.

Strip the intestine onto the viscera table with the knife. Make certain the small intestines hang out on the right side, to tense the mesentery. It is important when removing the small intestine, and indeed whenever cutting tissue, to maintain tension at all times (Fig. 7). The knife works more efficiently cutting tight tissue than loose tissue. Also, always keep the hand maintaining tension close to the knife hand. If the tensing hand is too far from the knife hand, decomposed intestine is more likely to tear. Whenever the knife is not being used, it should be fully sheathed in the nearest skeletal muscle. It should never be partially sheathed or dropped onto the table or into a body cavity. This should become a rigid habit; many nasty cuts will be avoided.

As the prosector comes to the ileal end of the small intestine, he should identify the ileocecal fold and transect the thick-walled ileum just proximal to the fold, leaving about 12 cm. of the ileum with the large intestine (Fig. 8).

If the small intestine is distended with gas or fluid, it may be difficult to displace it sufficiently to locate the duodenocolic fold. In this case simply pick up a loop of intestine at any point and strip it in both directions until the duodenal and ileal ends are identified.

After the small intestine has been removed, wash hands and steel the knife, observing the interior of the abdominal cavity (Fig. 9).

Gather up the great mesentery in the left hand, identify the lymph nodes in the root, and transect the root of the mesentery dorsal to the nodes. Remove the mesentery (Fig. 9).

Removal of the Large Intestine

Before removing the large intestine, isolate and examine the caudal mesenteric artery and ganglion together with the major nerve branches passing to the urogenital tract. They will be de-

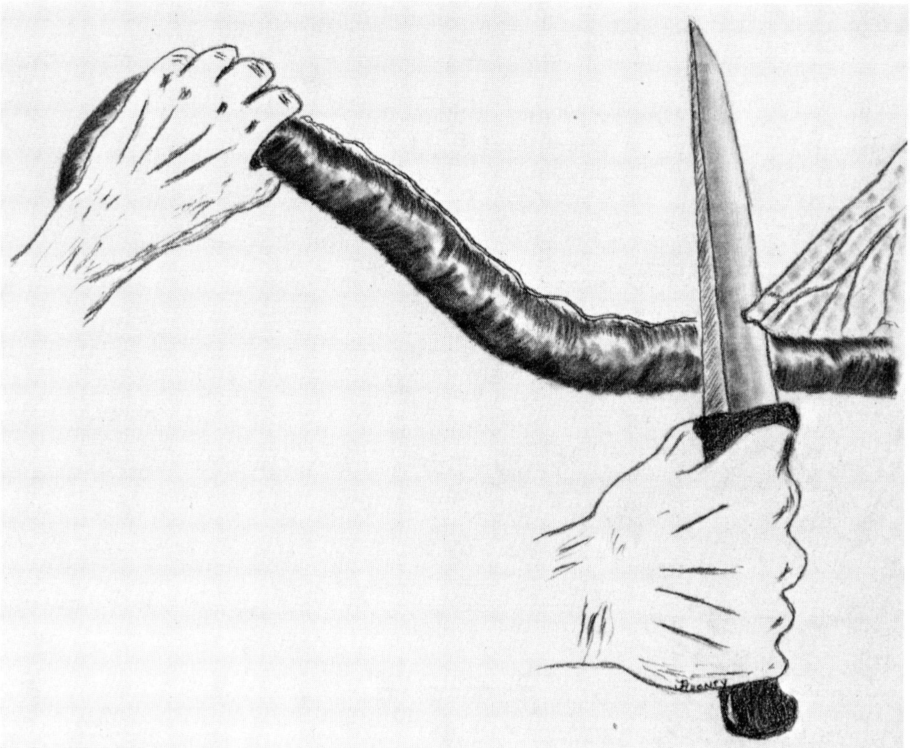

FIG. 7. Removing the small intestine by cutting it free from the mesentery.

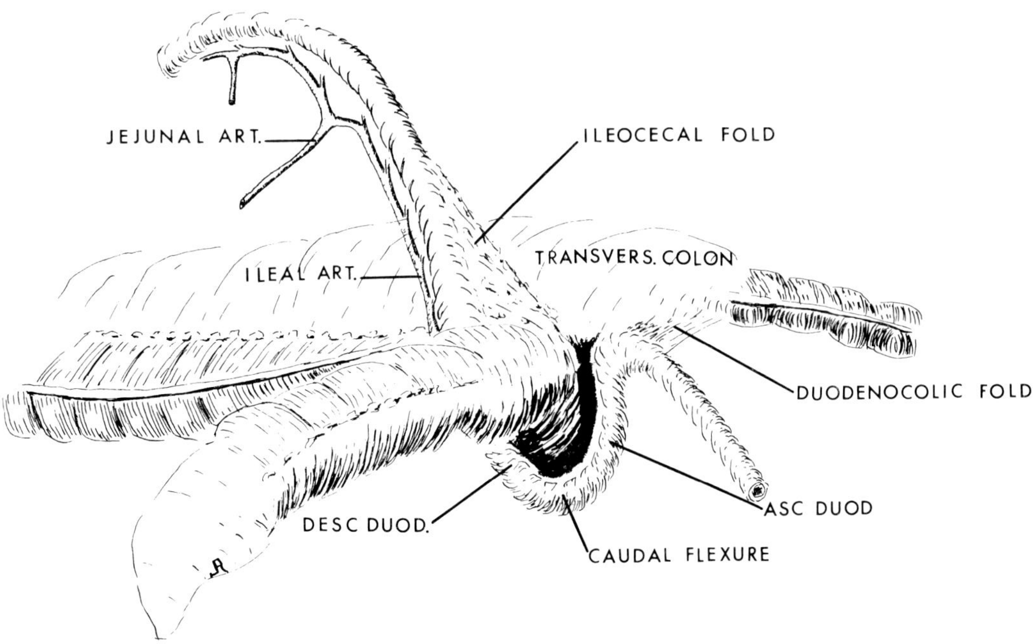

FIG. 8. The relationships of the ileocecal fold, duodenocolic fold, and caudal flexure of the duodenum. The end-to-end anastomosis of the ileal artery (branch of ileocecocolic artery) and the distal jejunal branch of the cranial mesenteric artery is also shown.

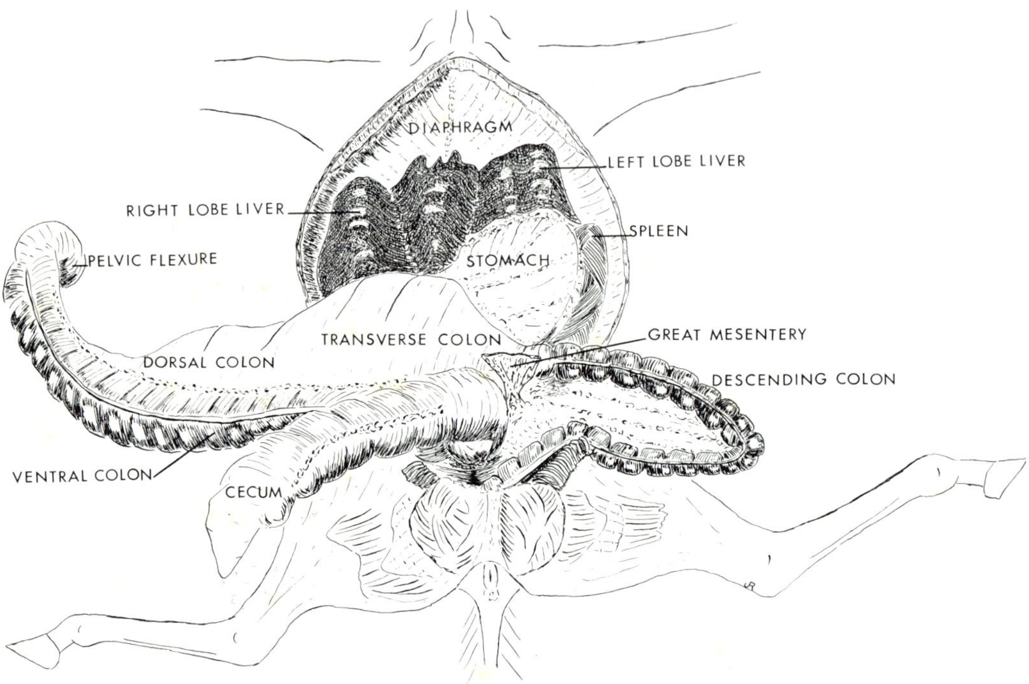

FIG. 9. Large colon and cecum displaced out the right side of the carcass and the descending colon out on the left. The small intestine has been removed.

stroyed during the subsequent dissection and must be examined now. Peel one-half of the mesocolon away and bluntly remove fat to expose the ganglion and its branches (Figs. 10 and 11).

Transect the descending colon at the junction with the rectum, approximately at the level of the pelvic inlet. Pull the descending colon to the right and strip it from the mesocolon, working proximally to the transverse colon. Gather up the mesocolon and remove it, cutting close to the origin from the sublumbar peritoneum.

Lift the greater omentum and note its attachment along the transverse colon. Break it loose from this attachment and lay it up over the stomach, out of the way of the ensuing dissection (Fig. 12).

Exerting steady, even traction with one hand, blunt dissect the transverse and right dorsal colon free from the left tail and body of the pancreas (Figs. 12 and 13). In the decomposed carcass care must be taken to avoid bursting the colon or mutilating the pancreas. The ventral surface of the portal vein will be exposed. Do not tear the vein.

Dissection of Cranial Mesenteric Artery

Palpate the area just caudal to the pancreas and to the right of the midline. The cranial mesenteric artery is felt as a hard, knobby cord (Fig. 14). Bluntly dissect around the artery until it can be completely encircled and held in the hand. Carefully strip down the artery to isolate the first 8 to 10 cm. of the branches of the ileocecocolic artery (ventral colic, dorsal colic, medial and lateral cecal arteries). The small middle colic artery which accompanies the descending colon may also be isolated, but it is quite small and is usually broken when the transverse colon is dissected free from the pancreas.

Transect the cranial mesenteric artery close to the aorta, so that it remains with the large intestine when the latter is removed. This is an undesirable blind cut since the origin of the ar-

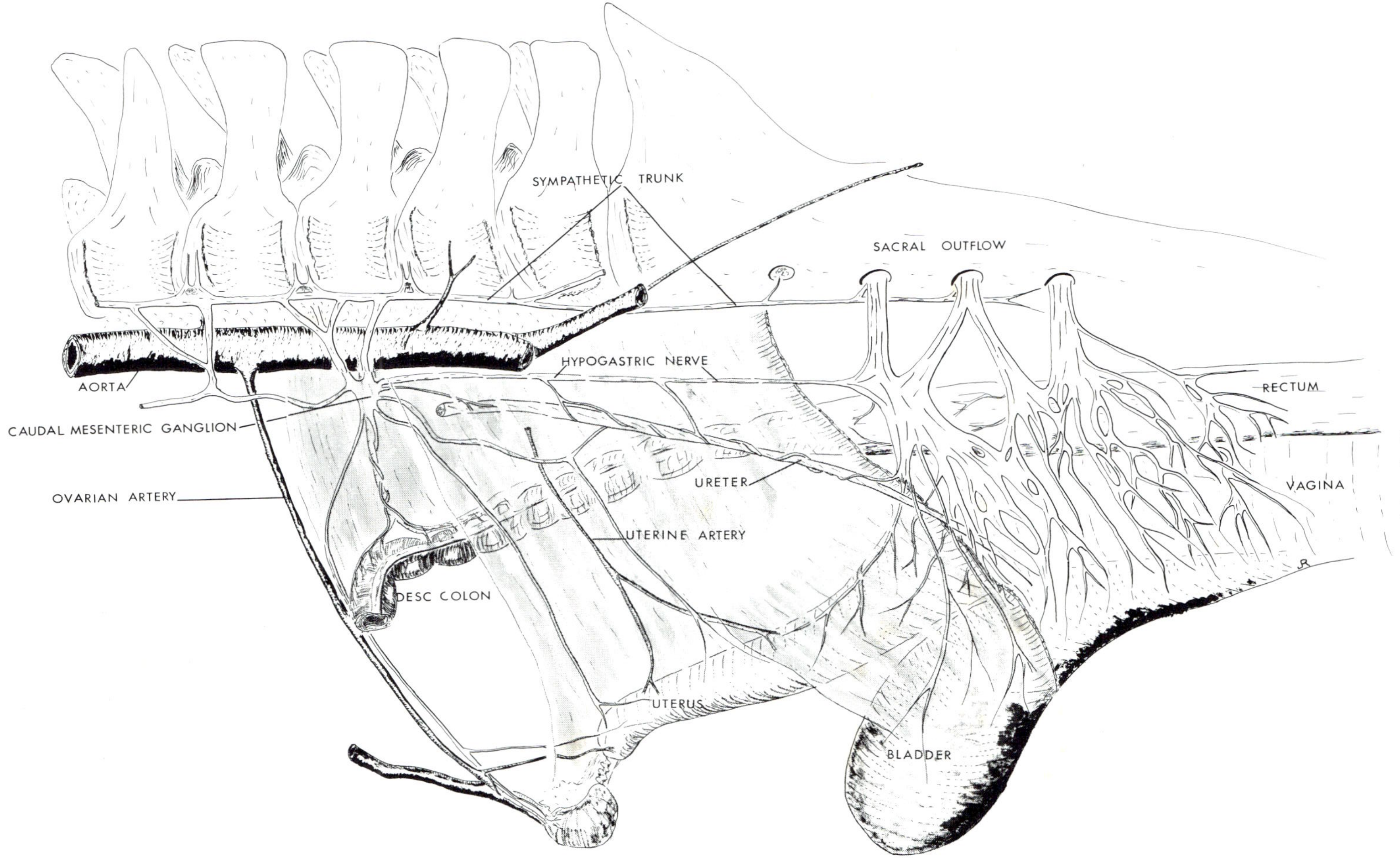

FIG. 10. Lateral view of the caudal mesenteric artery and ganglion and the autonomic nerves of the female pelvis.

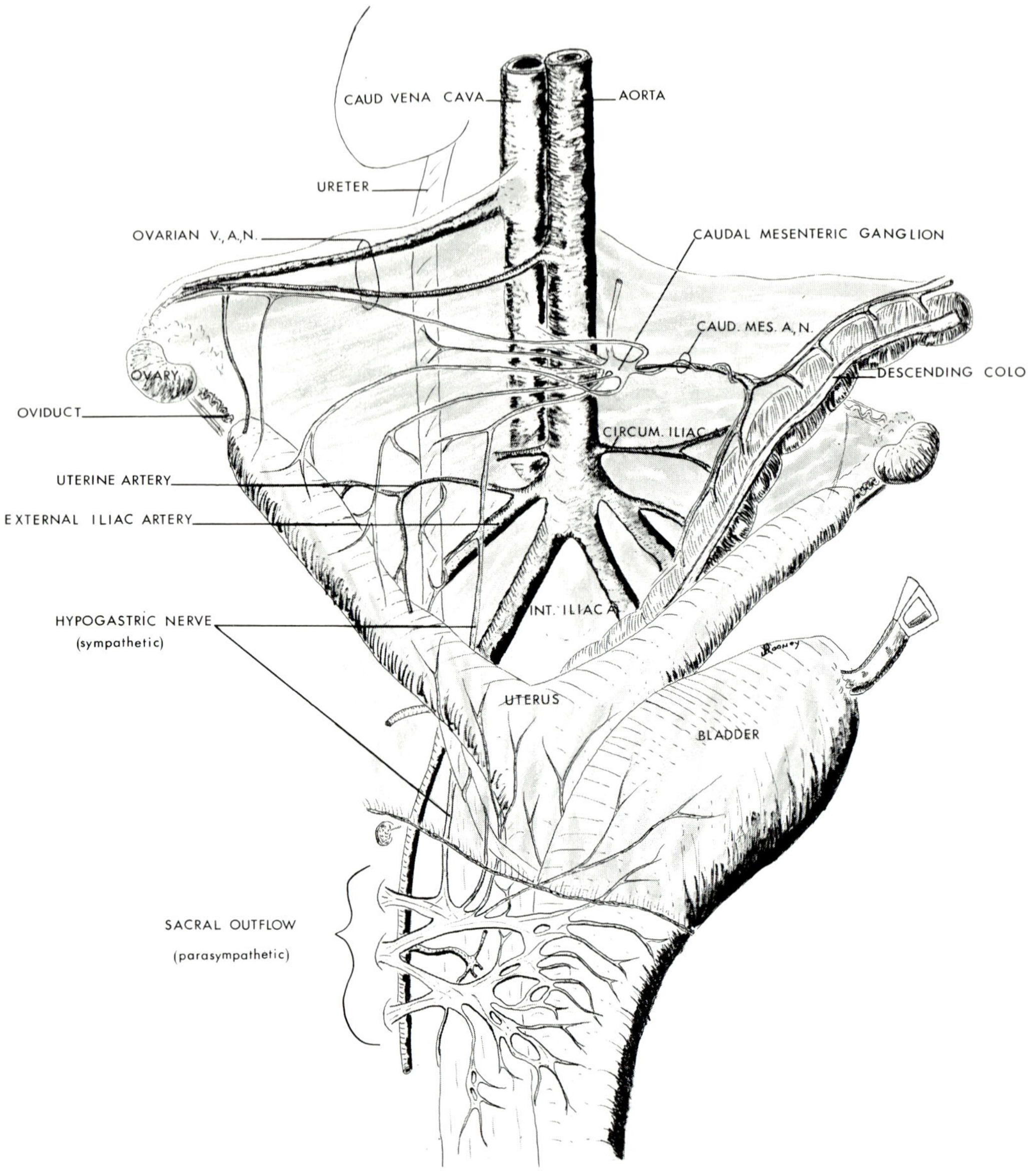

FIG. 11. Ventral view of Figure 10. The nerves are shown on one side only.

tery from the aorta cannot be clearly visualized. By laying the knife flat, however, unnecessary damage rarely occurs.

The large intestine is now held in place only by the areolar tissues between the head of the cecum and the sublumbar area. Exerting a continuous pull on the cecum and colon, bluntly dissect through this areolar tissue and roll the large intestine out on the table or ground. This dissection is easily accomplished; the prosector need only break down the tissues which are under tension as the large intestine pulls itself out of the abdominal cavity. The descending duodenum is attached by mesentery to the right dorsal colon. Break down this mesentery as the colon is removed, leaving the duodenum *in situ*.

Pause, rinse hands, and steel the knife,

examining the abdominal cavity. It is imperative to take these moments for examination and contemplation. The dissection must be anatomical; one must see everything possible before the next "layer" of tissues and organs is disturbed. At this level the stomach, the pylorus, and the whole of the descending duodenum are clearly visible, as is the pancreas, lying in the embrace of the duodenum (Fig. 14).

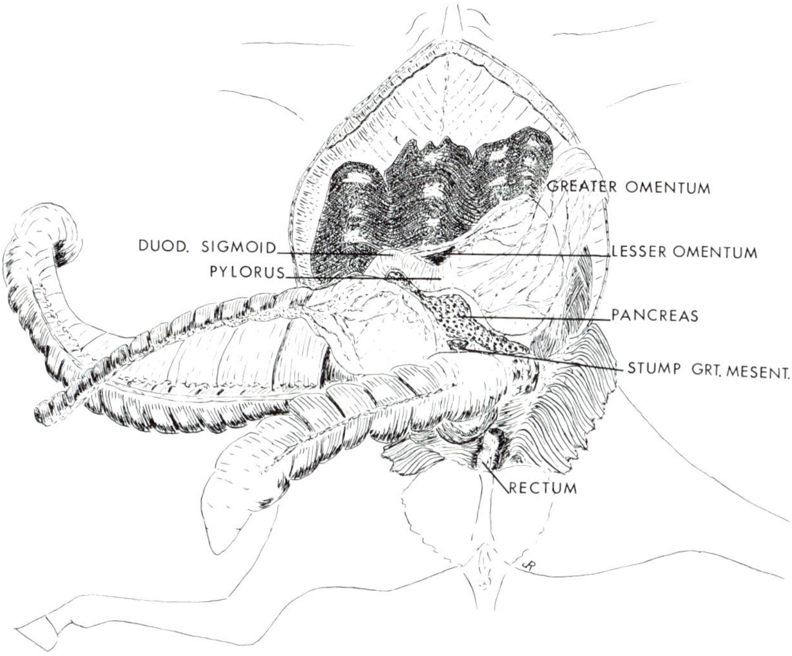

FIG. 12. The descending colon and transverse colon have been bluntly dissected from the pancreas and displaced to the right of the carcass. The left tail and body of the pancreas are exposed.

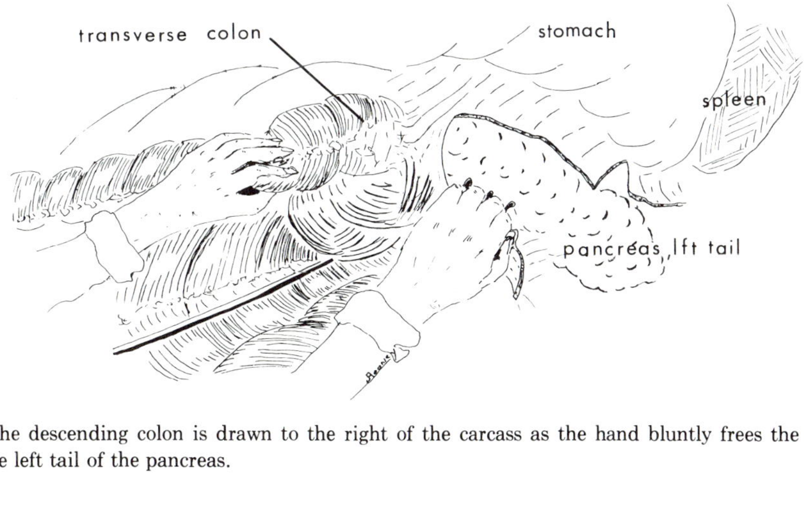

FIG. 13. The descending colon is drawn to the right of the carcass as the hand bluntly frees the transverse colon from the left tail of the pancreas.

Dissection of the Pancreas

With a spade-like motion of the hand, carefully blunt dissect the left tail of the pancreas free from the sublumbar attachments, starting at the left extremity and working toward the body of the pancreas, to the right. Scoop out the puddle of blood and palpate and blunt dissect the shorter right tail of the pancreas free from its sublumbar attachments. The left and right tails are now free (Fig. 15), and the head or body remains attached to the duodenum. The pancreas forms a ring around the portal vein. Sever or break the dorsal narrower part of the ring, being careful not to break the vein. The pancreatic ring is a convenient landmark for identification of the major trunk of the portal vein. With experience the prosector will note the portal vein and many of the branches much earlier in the dissection. It is clearly visible at this time.

I have never seen a significant lesion in the portal vein. However, the vein must be examined to avoid overlooking a significant lesion. Although I can say with cer-

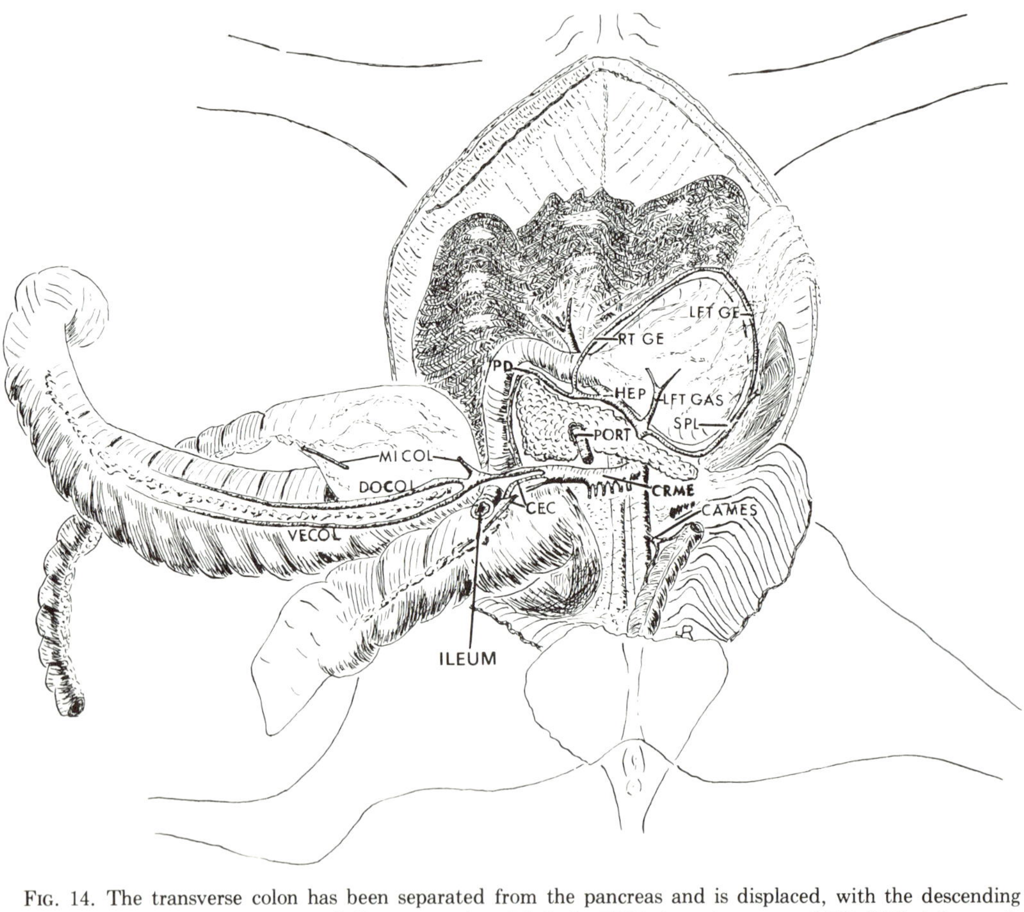

FIG. 14. The transverse colon has been separated from the pancreas and is displaced, with the descending colon, to the right of the carcass. Celiac artery (not labeled): *HEP*, hepatic artery; *LFT GAS*, left gastric artery; *SPL*, splenic artery; *LFT GE*, left gastroepiploic artery; *RT GE*, right gastroepiploic artery; *PD*, pancreaticoduodenal artery. Cranial mesenteric artery (*CRME*): *CEC*, medial and lateral cecal arteries; *MICOL*, middle colic artery, *DOCOL*, dorsal colic artery; *VECOL*, ventral colic artery. Caudal mesenteric artery, *CAMES;* portal vein, *PORT*.

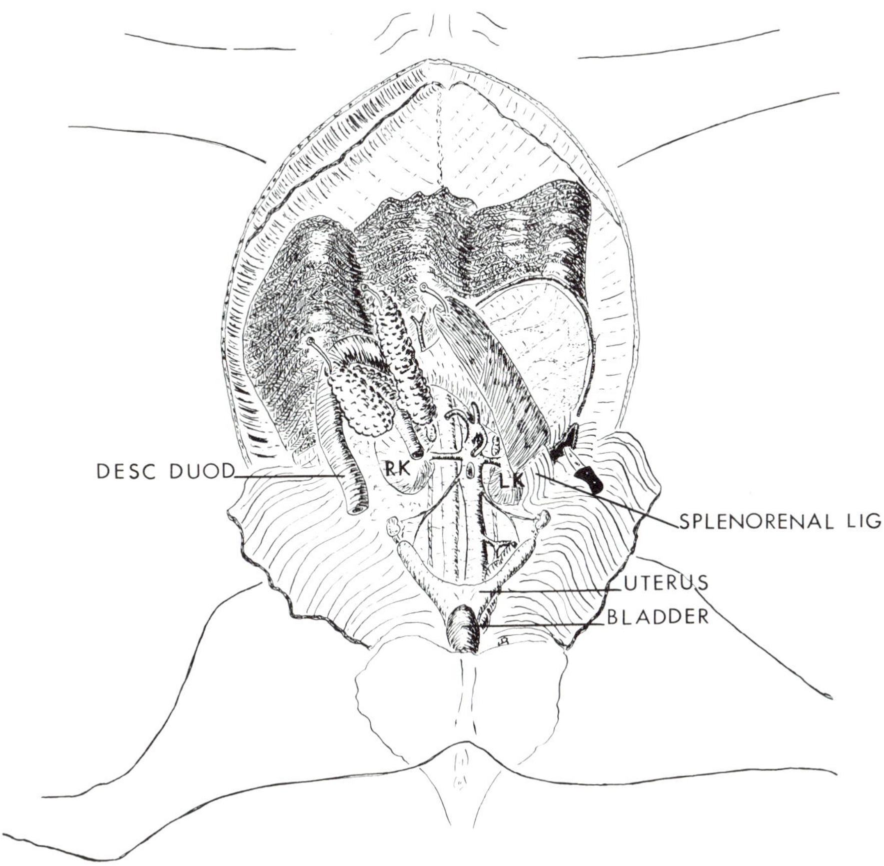

FIG. 15. The large intestine has been removed. The two tails of the pancreas, with the portal vein between, are held up for illustration. The tail of the spleen is pulled to the right and the knife is severing the splenorenal ligament. The transected stump of the cranial mesenteric artery (unlabeled) is shown just caudal to the celiac artery and its branches (unlabeled). *RK* and *LK*: right and left kidneys.

tainty after many thousand autopsies that lesions of the portal vein are extremely rare, that very simple fact would not be known if the vein had never been examined.

Dissection of the Celiac Artery

Examine the V-shaped space between the caudal edge of the left tail of the pancreas and the duodenum over (ventral to) the caudal vena cava (which is just dorsal to the portal vein). The hepatic branch of the celiac artery is both visible and palpable (Fig. 14). Strip this artery close to the portal area of the liver and transect it close to the liver. Move the hand to the left and pick up the left gastric branch of the celiac before it fans out on the visceral surface of the stomach. Strip the artery and transect it close to the first branching on the stomach. Continue to the left into the space between the stomach, left kidney, and spleen and pick up the large splenic artery, the last branch of the celiac. Strip it to the spleen (about 12 cm.) and transect at the spleen. Since the liver, spleen, and stomach must be removed separately, the transection is not close to the aorta as with the cranial mesenteric artery.

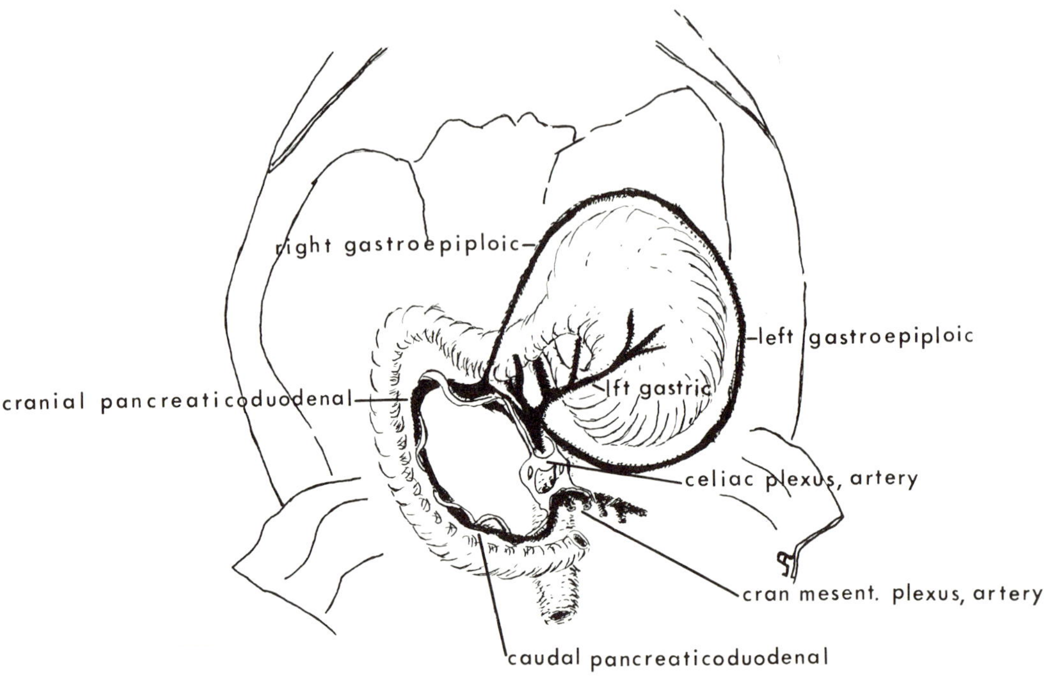

FIG. 16. The arterial supply of the stomach and descending duodenum. The cranial (branch of celiac a) and caudal (branch of cranial mesenteric a) pancreaticoduodenal arteries anastomose end-to-end. Nerves accompany all the vessels but are shown only for the pancreaticoduodenal.

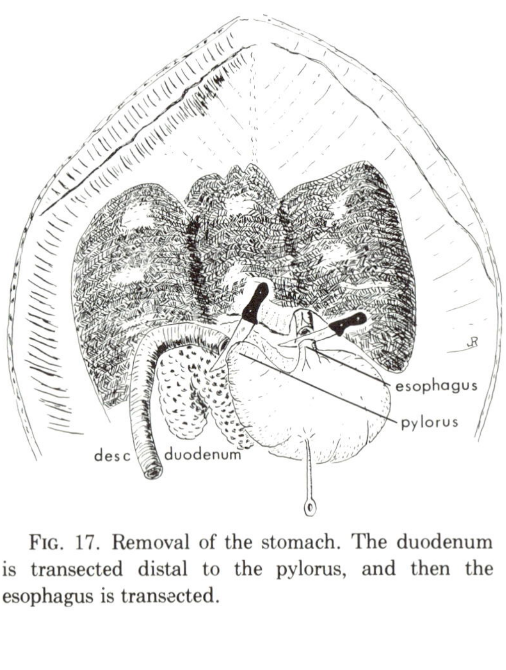

FIG. 17. Removal of the stomach. The duodenum is transected distal to the pylorus, and then the esophagus is transected.

The above procedure is routine. One should, before stripping these vessels, closely observe their course and relationships. The autonomic nerves from the celiac ganglia accompany the vessels and are readily palpated, seen, and examined. In acute gastric dilatation the pancreaticoduodenal branches of the hepatic artery should be examined with care. Lesions in either the nerves or the vessels of the descending duodenum could help to explain otherwise idiopathic cases of acute gastric dilatation (Fig. 16).

Removal of the Spleen

Pull the tail of the spleen to the right and locate the splenorenal ligament. Sever the ligament and draw the spleen to the right, cutting the gastrosplenic ligament, and remove the

spleen, gastrosplenic ligament, and greater omentum as a unit (Fig. 15).

Removal of the Stomach

Draw the duodenum and stomach caudad and identify the lesser omentum between the stomach, duodenum, and liver. Break through the lesser omentum with the fingers, running the hand underneath the duodenum and breaking through (from the dorsal side). Palpate the firm pylorus and transect the duodenum just distal to the pylorus. Continuing to draw the stomach caudad and toward the right side, isolate and transect the intra-abdominal portion of the esophagus. Break down the gastrophrenic ligament and loose areolar tissue between the dorsal part of the greater curvature of the stomach and the crura of the diaphragm by blunt dissection. Remove the stomach (Fig. 17).

Removal of the Liver, Pancreas, and Descending Duodenum

Sever the right triangular ligament of the liver for about 8 cm., tensing the ligament by

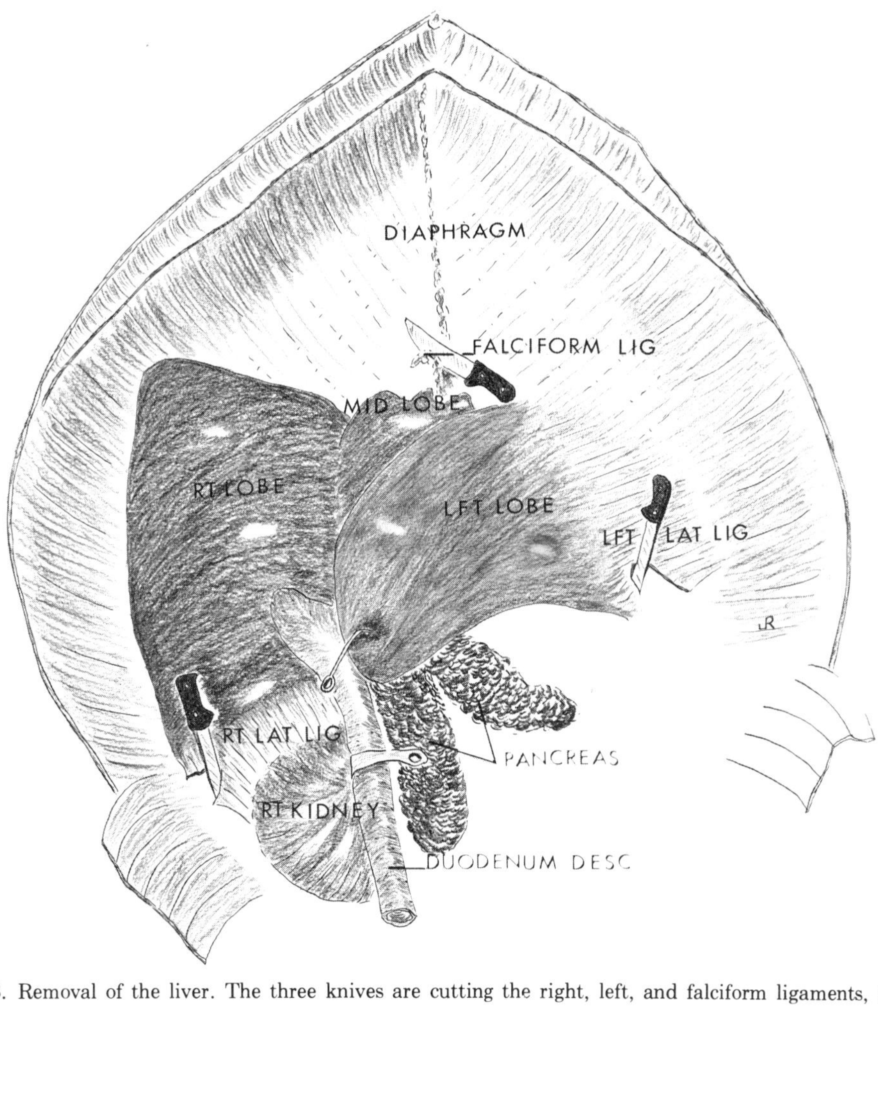

FIG. 18. Removal of the liver. The three knives are cutting the right, left, and falciform ligaments, in that order.

lifting the right lobe and displacing it toward the left (Fig. 18). Sheath the knife in muscle and insert the left hand under (dorsal to) the liver to the midline, palpating the hepatorenal ligament between the caudate lobe of the liver and the right kidney. At the midline a small pocket or pouch may be encountered. Drive two or more fingers firmly into this pouch, tearing the ligament. If the pouch is not apparent, simply break through the ligament at this point. Be sure that the fingers are showing between the caudate lobe of the liver and the right kidney. Draw the hand laterally to the right, tearing the ligament to join the previously severed outer edge (Fig. 19). The process may have to be repeated several times. The initial knife cut in the ligament is necessary because the lateral part of the ligament is quite heavy, difficult to tear, and can bruise or cut the hand.

Pull the left lobe of the liver to the right (Fig. 18) and sever the left triangular ligament to or near to the midline. There may be fibrous adhesions (perihepatitis filamentosa), particularly between the left lobe of the liver and the diaphragm. Note their position and break them down carefully in order to proceed with the dissection.

Draw the entire liver caudad and to the right and sever the falciform ligament, continuing the incision into but not through the caudal vena cava. Keep this incision close to the liver to avoid cutting the diaphragm. Introduce two fingers into the vena cava and tear it open through the left wall (Fig. 20). It is necessary to nick the palpable firm ring before the vena cava can be split. Examine the lining of the vena cava.

Insert a finger of the left hand into the large orifice of the hepatic vein of the left lobe, as a handhold, and draw the liver out on the right side. Sever the right wall of the vena cava, freeing the liver (Fig. 20). If this is properly done, one-half of the vena cava will remain in the carcass and one-half will be with the liver. Often, the liver will be torn slightly. Do not be concerned. Transect the vena cava at the caudal end of the initial finger-splitting incision and remove

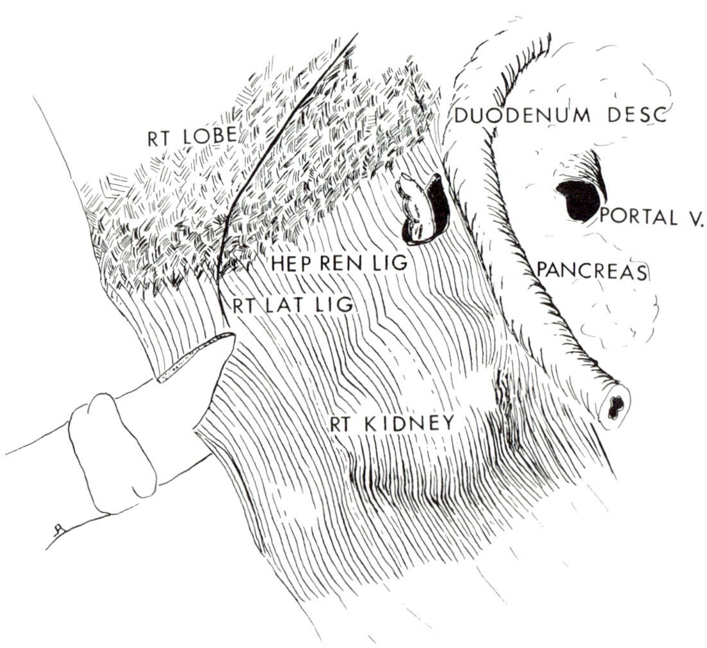

FIG. 19. Detail of tearing out the ligament between the right kidney and the caudate lobe of the liver (hepatorenal ligament) to join the initial knife incision in the right lateral ligament.

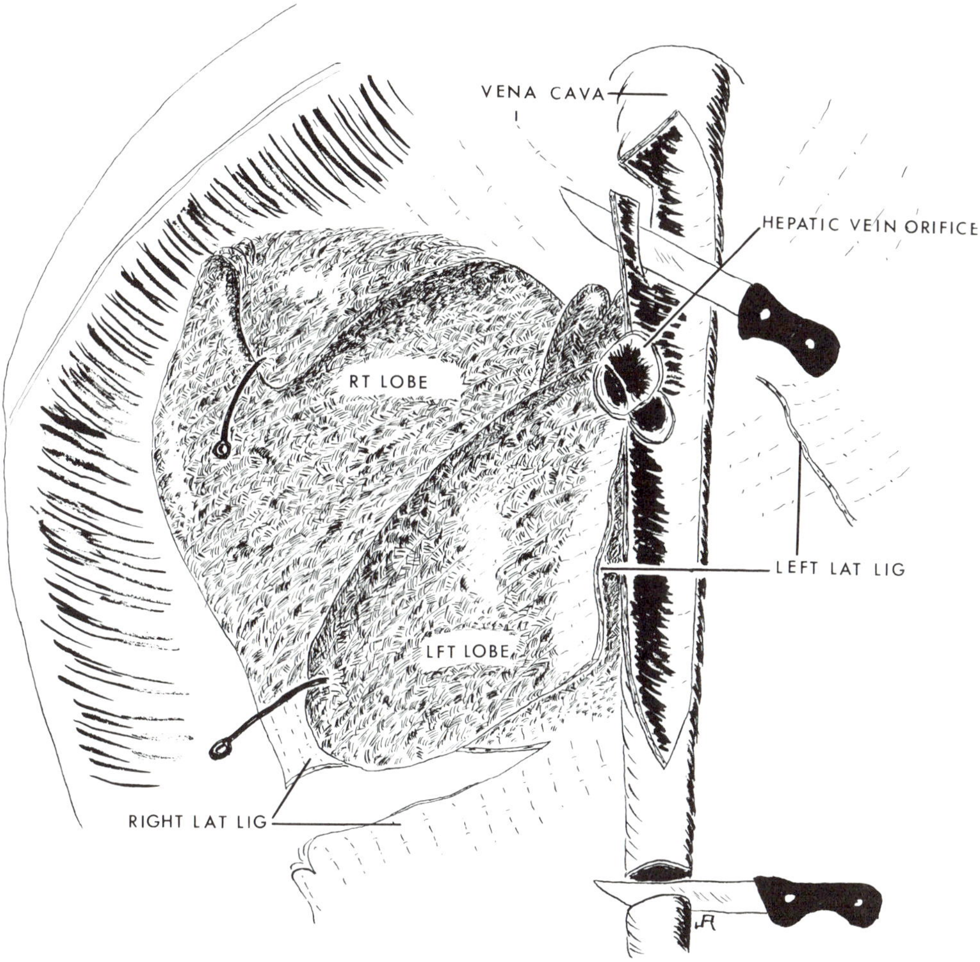

FIG. 20. Removal of the liver. The right lateral (triangular) ligament and hepatorenal ligament have been cut and torn out. The left lateral (triangular) ligament and falciform ligament have been severed, and the caudal vena cava torn open. The upper knife is cutting through the wall of the vena cava as the liver is drawn out on the right side of the carcass. The lower knife is transecting the vena cava (this would, in fact, be done after the liver had been drawn almost completely out of the carcass).

the liver, pancreas, and descending duodenum *en bloc*.

Pause, steel the knife, and contemplate. Is the diaphragm tense and convex or bulged backward? In the latter case pleuritis or pneumothorax may be suspected. Although pneumothorax is not common in horses, the diagnosis will be made only by noting at this time a loose diaphragm with no exudate or effusion when the diaphragm is removed. One may complain that, since pneumothorax is rare, why bother? The answer is simple: the easy diagnosis can be made by anyone, with any style of autopsy procedure; the difficult, unusual, and very satisfying diagnosis will be made only by the discerning prosector utilizing a systematic, anatomical autopsy procedure.

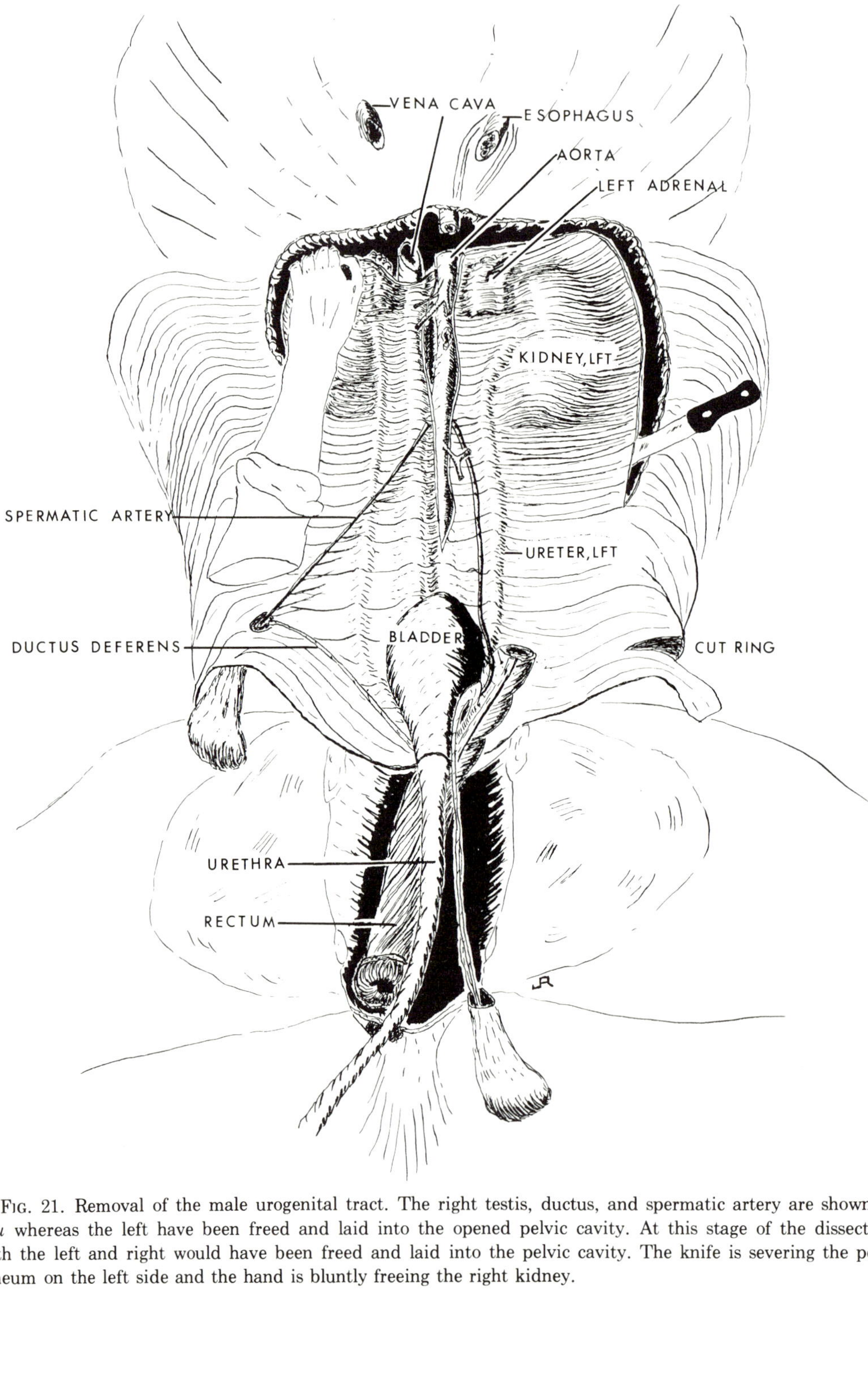

FIG. 21. Removal of the male urogenital tract. The right testis, ductus, and spermatic artery are shown *in situ* whereas the left have been freed and laid into the opened pelvic cavity. At this stage of the dissection both the left and right would have been freed and laid into the pelvic cavity. The knife is severing the peritoneum on the left side and the hand is bluntly freeing the right kidney.

Removal of the Urogenital Tract and Rectum

Remove the muscle from the ventral surface of the pelvis and remove a central block of bone by sagittal, parallel saw cuts passing through the pubis, obturator foramina and ischium. When sawing concentrate on the pubis first, with the saw blade directed dorsomedially. The blade tends to cut laterally, and this is counteracted by directing it medially at the start. When the pubis has been sawed through, concentrate on the ischium. If one attempts to saw both at the same time, the blade will frequently go awry. If the animal is on the table and the hip joints have not been opened, one cut may be made and, by sharply, briskly pushing down on the legs, the pelvic cavity will be opened sufficiently. This works particularly well in older animals and postparturient mares. In effect the sacroiliac joint and ligaments are disrupted, allowing the pelvis to open. If one wishes to examine the sacroiliac area (obscure rearleg lameness), the block of bone should be removed and no pressure exerted to open the pelvis. In foals the cartilagenous symphysis pubis is readily split with a knife.

In the male, the penis must be freed from the symphysis and ischial arch by severing the suspensory ligaments and crura, if not done earlier. The penis should be left in continuity with the intrapelvic viscera. Free the anus and penis or anus and vulva by a semicircular incision in the perineal region.

Lay the testis, ductus, etc. into the pelvic cavity so that they will not be cut off inadvertently.

Incise the peritoneum cranial to the left kidney and adrenal gland, continuing the incision parallel and lateral to the lateral border of the kidney and lateral to the ureter and uterine horn to the pelvic inlet (Fig. 21).

Repeat on the right side. To avoid puncturing the diaphragm it is advisable to blunt dissect the right kidney and adrenal from their sublumbar attachments and then incise the peritoneum to the pelvic inlet as on the left side.

Locate the branches of the celiac artery and transect the aorta just cranial to the celiac artery. Continue the incision to the ventral surface of the vertebrae. Gathering both kidneys in one hand, draw them caudad and, with the knife lying flat in the frontal plane, free the entire mass of sublumbar viscera—kidneys, adrenals, aorta, vena cava, ureters, rectum, and reproductive organs—from the carcass. Continue the reflection through the pelvic cavity, being careful to include the testes, ductus, etc., until the entire mass is freed and removed. When reflecting through the pelvis, first draw the viscera to one side and lay the knife cut between the viscera and the wall of the pelvic cavity. Then draw the viscera to the opposite side and cut on the other side. Although the knife should be in the frontal plane during reflection from the sublumbar area, it should be almost sagittal when reflecting through the pelvic cavity. These instructions are given to avoid cutting the visceral mass into two parts and to facilitate the removal.

Locate and open the external and internal iliac arteries. They were cut off close to the pelvic inlet as the urogenital block was being removed.

The external iliac artery or one of the several branches of the internal iliac artery may rupture during parturition and result in fatal postpartum hemorrhage (80). The intimal surface of the external iliac is normally somewhat corrugated.

Slice the iliopsoas muscles and examine the cut surfaces. Remove the iliopsoas and the connective tissue covering the ventrocaudal aspect of the sacroiliac joints. They are lateral to and approximately in the same transverse plane as the lumbosacral articulation (prominent bump). If the pelvis has been "sprung" open as described earlier, one or both joints will be broken open. Examine the ventrocaudal sacroiliac ligaments.

THREE

Evisceration of the Thorax, Neck, and Head

Dissection

Dissection of the Diaphragm

Incise the diaphragm along the costal insertion on either the left or right side, not on the midline. Note the collapse or loosening of the diaphragm on that side. In some horses the opposite side of the diaphragm collapses immediately because of an incomplete mediastinum. In other horses it may collapse after a few minutes presumably because the loose mediastinum shifts. In the remaining cases the mediastinum is complete and the opposite side does not collapse.

Insert the hand through the incision and palpate the caudal mediastinum. Break down the mediastinum. Pull the diaphragm down and back and continue the incision around both sides. Sever the caudal vena cava and the phrenic nerves, and free the thoracic portion of the esophagus and the aorta from the diaphragmatic hiatuses so that the diaphragm may be completely laid down. Run the hand forward, along one side of the heart, until the cranial mediastinum can be palpated and broken down. Draw the hand strongly up and back, breaking down the sternal attachment of the pericardium and dropping the heart down. Try not to tear open the pericardium.

Examine the pleural cavity, noting adhesions which may be destroyed during the removal of the thoracic viscera. There are normally about 100 ml. of clear yellow fluid in each pleural cavity.

Dissection of the Thoracic Viscera, Neck, and Throat

Two different procedures are employed for the removal of the heart and lungs, depending upon the age of the animal.

1. In the foal remove the sternum by severing the costal cartilages on both sides with the knife. The point of the knife must be directed laterally, outward, to avoid cutting the pericardium and heart. The knife is inserted from inside out about midway and pulled back, severing the cartilages. It is then directed forward to cut the remaining cartilages. Repeat on the opposite side (Fig. 22).

2. In the adult the sternum is not removed, and the heart and lungs will be removed as follows: Reflect the skin from the ventral surface of the cranial and cervical regions if not already done. (*Be careful to note the mandibular lymph nodes. They should not be removed with the skin.*)

Slice on either side of the larynx, carrying the incisions boldly and deeply forward just inside the rami of the mandible and lateral to the tongue as far forward as possible. Unite the two incisions transversely in the angulus mentalis. As the knife is brought forward past the larynx, it may encounter resistance from the hyoid bones. Do not try to overcome this resistance; simply allow the knife to ride over the bones and continue rostrally.

Draw the tongue caudad out through the mandibular space using the knife to free the rostral end. Sever the soft palate transversely

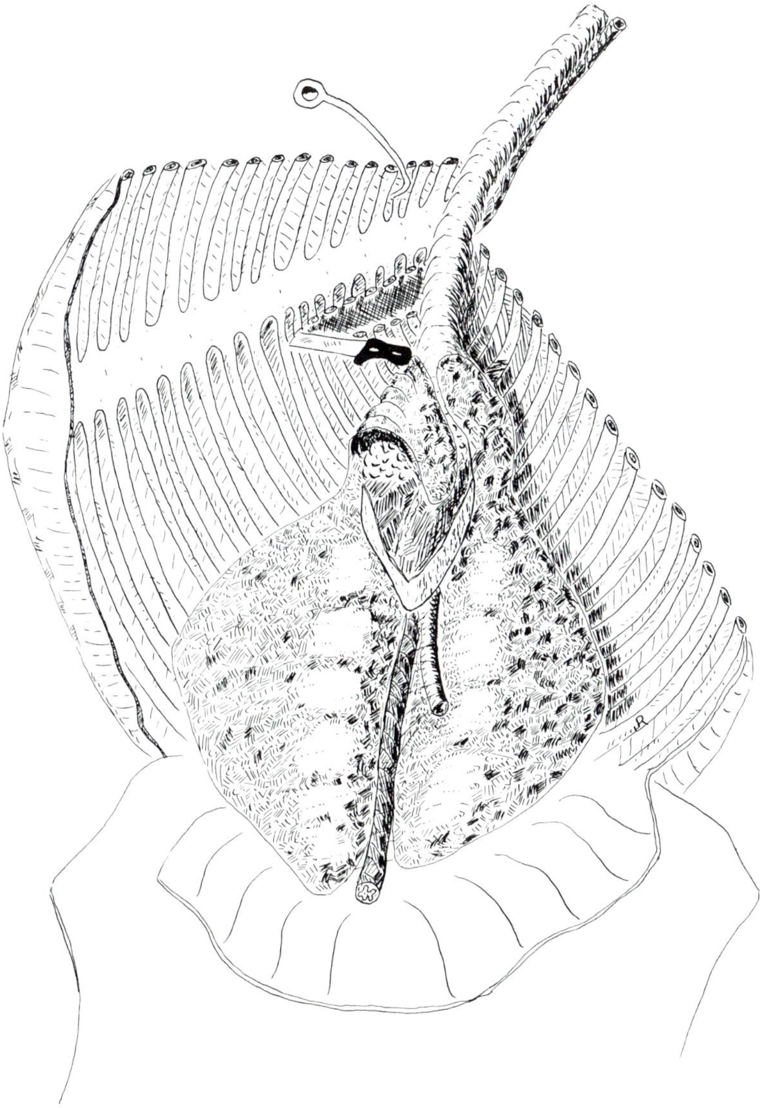

FIG. 22. Removal of the sternum in the foal. The pericardium is shown partially removed, and the aorta and esophagus are shown. In fact, the pericardium is not opened until later and the esophagus and aorta would not be visible at this stage.

and free the dorsal wall of the pharynx by traction on the tongue. The objective is to remove the entire pharyngeal ring intact (Fig. 23).

Palpate the stylohyoids (great cornua) and keratohyoids (small cornua) and insert the knife, with the edge rostrad, into the angle between them. Resting the tip of the knife on the hard palate or against the inside of the mandible, sever each articulation. As the soft palate is cut and the tongue is pulled back, one or both of the great cornua may be broken. This should be avoided if possible, but if it does occur, beware of the broken bone ends.

Continuing tension on the tongue, free the larynx, trachea and esophagus to the thoracic inlet, keeping the jugular veins, carotid arteries,

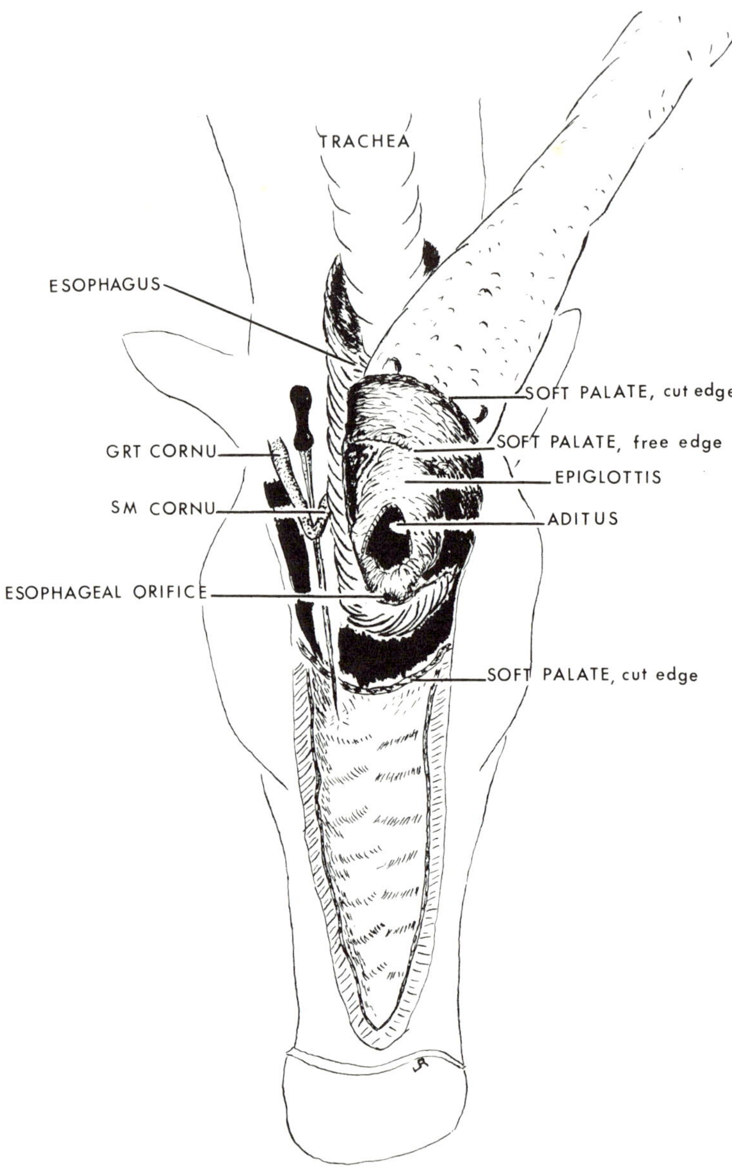

FIG. 23. Removal of the tongue and pharynx. The knife is severing the articulation between the great and small cornua.

vagosympathetic nerves, and recurrent nerves with the trachea and esophagus.

In the young animal, with the sternum removed, sever the vessels and nerves in the thoracic inlet by parallel knife cuts just inside the first ribs. With steady traction on the tongue, the cervical and thoracic viscera may be removed *en bloc*.

In the adult transect the cervical viscera (trachea, esophagus, etc.) in the midcervical region. Open the thoracic inlet by a circular incision just inside the first ribs and manubrium

sterni. Introduce the cut ends of the trachea and esophagus through the thoracic inlet into the thoracic cavity. A small incision between two tracheal rings provides a convenient handhold.

Within the thoracic cavity, grasp the trachea and steadily draw the thoracic viscera out of the cavity (Fig. 24). One hand has the handhold while the other hand grasps the trachea close to the base of the heart. A minimum of further sharp dissection may be necessary, particularly on the left side, in order to free the structures in the thoracic inlet.

Removing the Head

Remove the head by exerting strong dorsiflexion (over the edge of the table, a block of wood, or some other fulcrum) and transecting the rectus capitus ventralis muscle as it widens over the atlanto-occipital joint. Continue the incision into the spinal canal and transect the spinal cord. The atlanto-occipital joints should be opened with the knife edge directed craniolaterally (Fig. 25) to avoid sawing away on the bone.

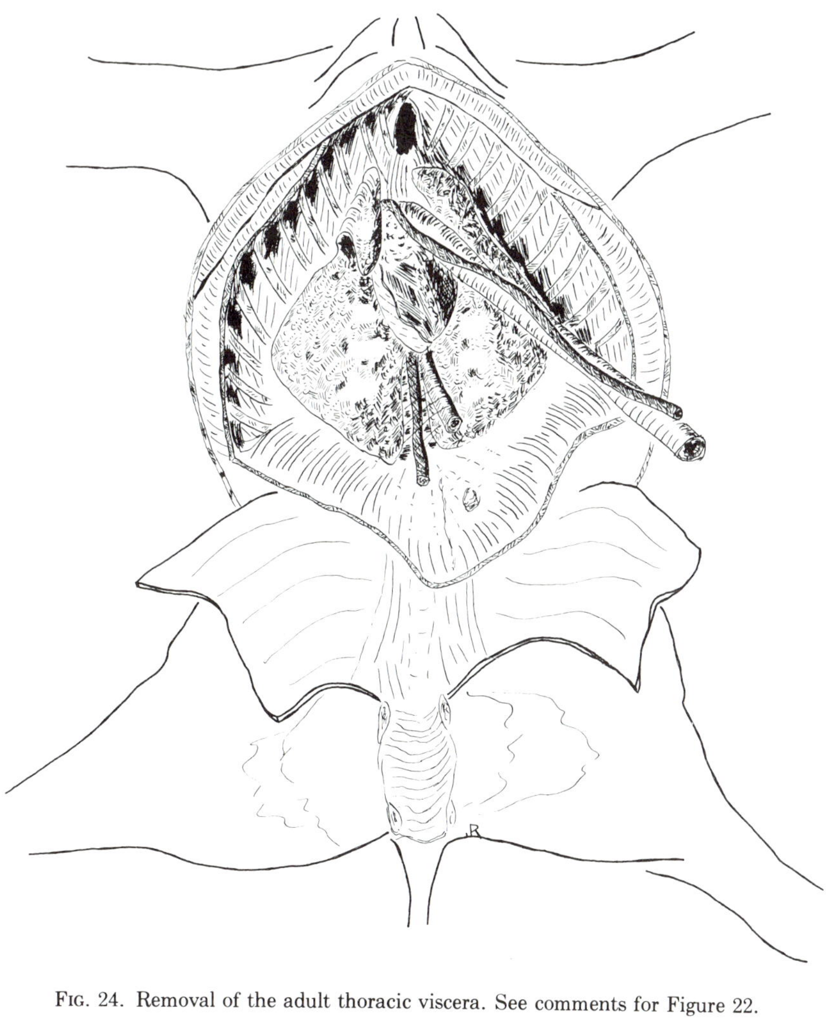

FIG. 24. Removal of the adult thoracic viscera. See comments for Figure 22.

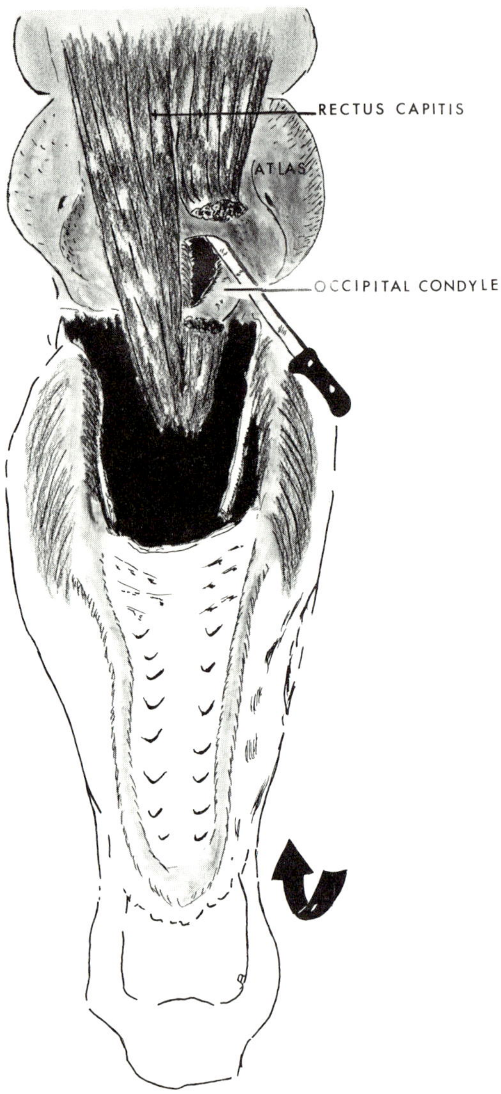

FIG. 25. Removal of the head. In fact, the rectus capitus muscle would be completely transected, as would the spinal cord, before opening the atlanto-occipital joint.

Interpretation

Examine the exposed portions of the head, neck, and chest. The mandibular lymph nodes are readily examined. The retropharyngeal lymph nodes were exposed as the throat viscera were drawn back. These nodes may be enlarged, hyperemic, and edematous in cases of acute upper respiratory disease. In strangles they may be enlarged, hard, fibrous abscesses with a creamy, purulent content.

The parotid lymph node and salivary glands will be examined later.

The guttural pouches will have been opened. Empyema or *Luftsackstein* (inspissated balls of pus) should be noted and cultured if present. (The pouches will be discussed in more detail below.)

The massive fibrinous and fibrofibrinous exudates and fluids characteristic of streptococcal pleuritis do not require extensive comment (Fig. 26). It may be well to note at this point, however, that a thorough search of the lung for an abscess must subsequently be made. Virtually every case of pleuritis arises from a focal abscess or abscesses in the lung. Occasionally a few fibrous strands may stretch from the parietal pleura to the lung. It is reasonable to assume that these are remnants of a healed pleuritis.

Rib fractures are not uncommon in newborn foals. The great majority are costochondral separations of no clinical significance. Fractures of the middle third of one or more ribs frequently accompany difficult parturition and sometimes normal parturition. The fracture ends may traumatize the lung and/or heart and may, rarely, damage soft tissue sufficiently to cause fatal hemorrhage or pneumothorax (tearing of lung or skin). It may be suggested that such fractures occur during parturition because of inadequate extension of the forelegs with the elbows jamming against the ribs. The majority of such fractures involve the ribs at the level of the elbow (35).

When the head is removed, the dura incised, and the atlanto-occipital joint

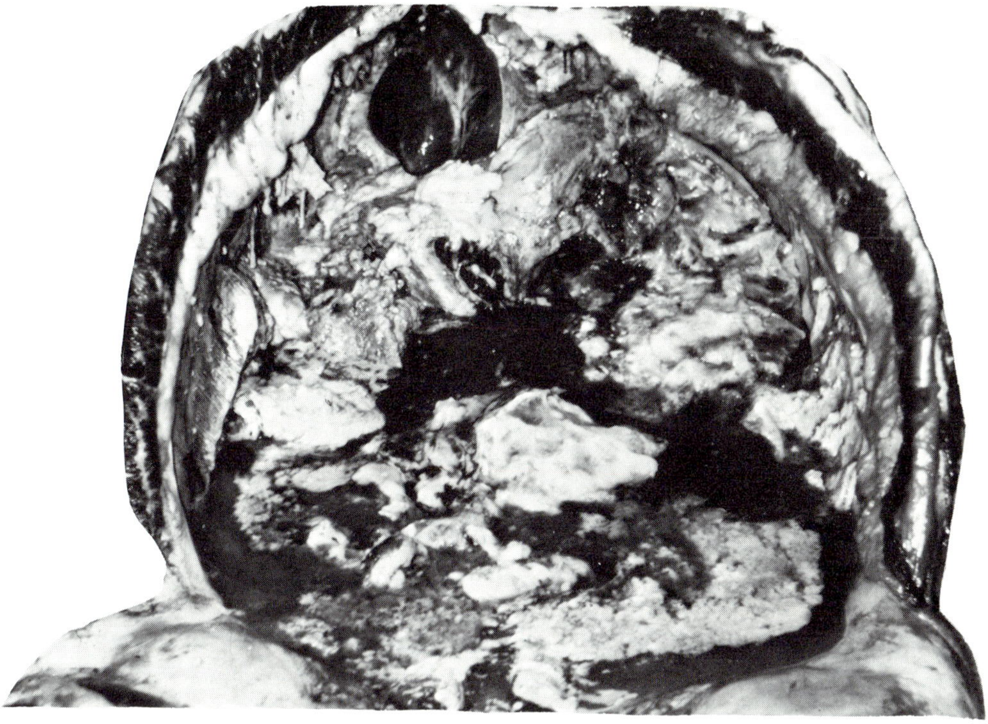

FIG. 26. Massive fibrinopurulent pleuritis. The heart is apparent at the upper left. The lungs are completely obscured by fibrin (white in photo) and "rivers" of purulent exudate (dark in photo).

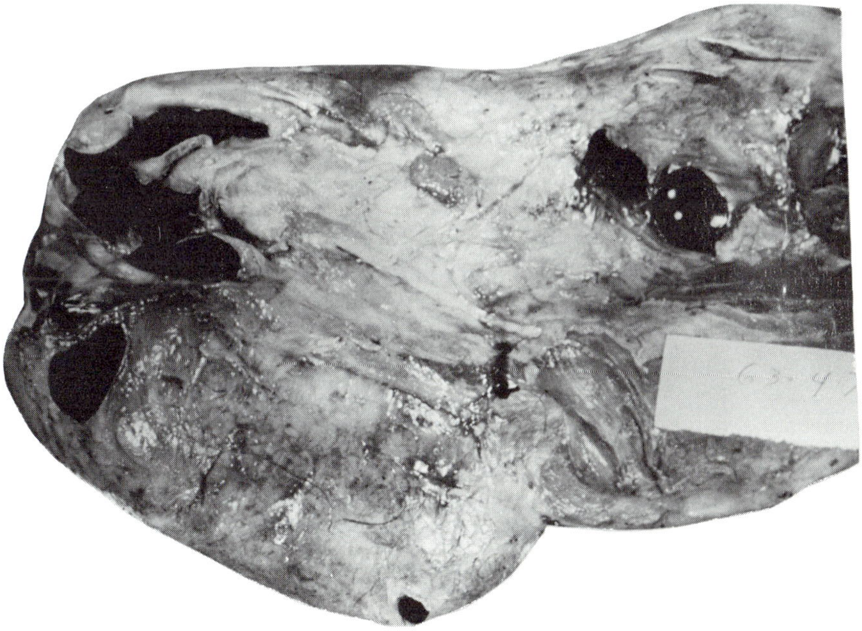

FIG. 27. Odontogenic cyst of the mandible of a newborn foal.

opened, a quantity of synovial fluid, cerebrospinal fluid, and blood from the longitudinal venous sinuses invariably pours out. No determination of increased cerebrospinal fluid quantity or pressure should be made. If cerebrospinal fluid is to be examined, the cisterna magna may be punctured from the dorsal side before the head is removed.

Odontogenic cysts are seen with some frequency particularly in the mandible, but also in the maxilla (Fig. 27), of young horses (102). They may be apparent at birth or become apparant through enlargement after birth. Although there is dispute about nomenclature (other names: adamantinoma, mucous cyst) and pathology, these appear to be congenital malformations of the permanent teeth primordia.

"Big head," or nutritional secondary hyperparathyroidism, occurs in horses. The condition has been thoroughly described in a recent report (55). It should not be confused with odontogenic cyst.

A variety of congenital defects of the several components of the teeth have been described in horses: hypoplasia of invaginated enamel and hypoplasia of infundibular cementum, for example (16). Certain of these defects are said to predispose to caries.

FOUR

The Locomotor System

In this chapter only a bare outline of locomotor lesions can be presented. Such lesions have been discussed in detail elsewhere (84).

Throughout the examination of the musculoskeletal system the prosector must continuously utilize his eyes and fingers, to detect abnormalities. Specific mention will not be made of nerves and vessels, but they should be noted carefully as the dissection proceeds (70). Bones, also, are not described in detail, but it is understood that they will be palpated whenever possible and carefully fleshed out where lesions are suspected. The skin should be removed completely from the area of a joint or other deep structure before dissecting. If the animal has been hoisted or dragged by either chains or ropes around the legs, rather startling postmortem bruising and distortion of structure may be present.

The following general rules should always be follwed when the legs are being dissected: (1) stand as shown in Figure 28; (2) keep both hands distal to the part being dissected; (3) use one hand to push downward on the distal end of the part being dissected; (4) in so far as possible have the knife tip pointing away from the prosector. If these rules are followed, the technique for opening the joints will be quickly mastered and the danger of inadvertent cuts will be minimized.

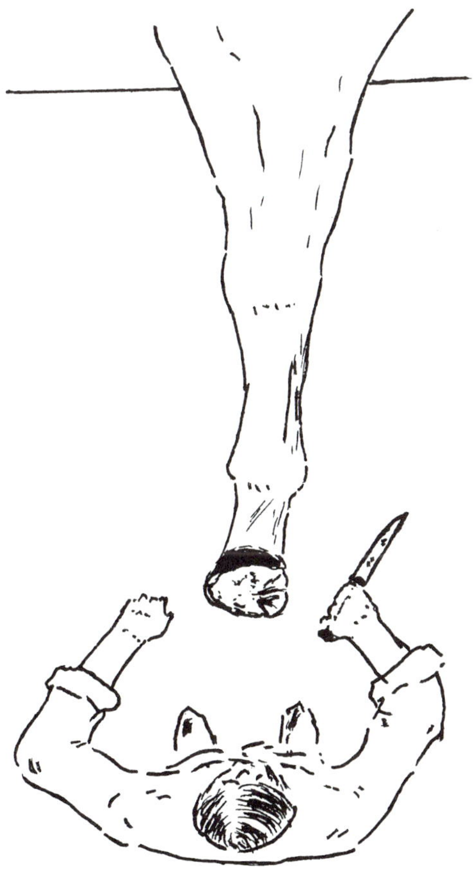

FIG. 28. Position of prosector when dissecting the legs, fore and rear.

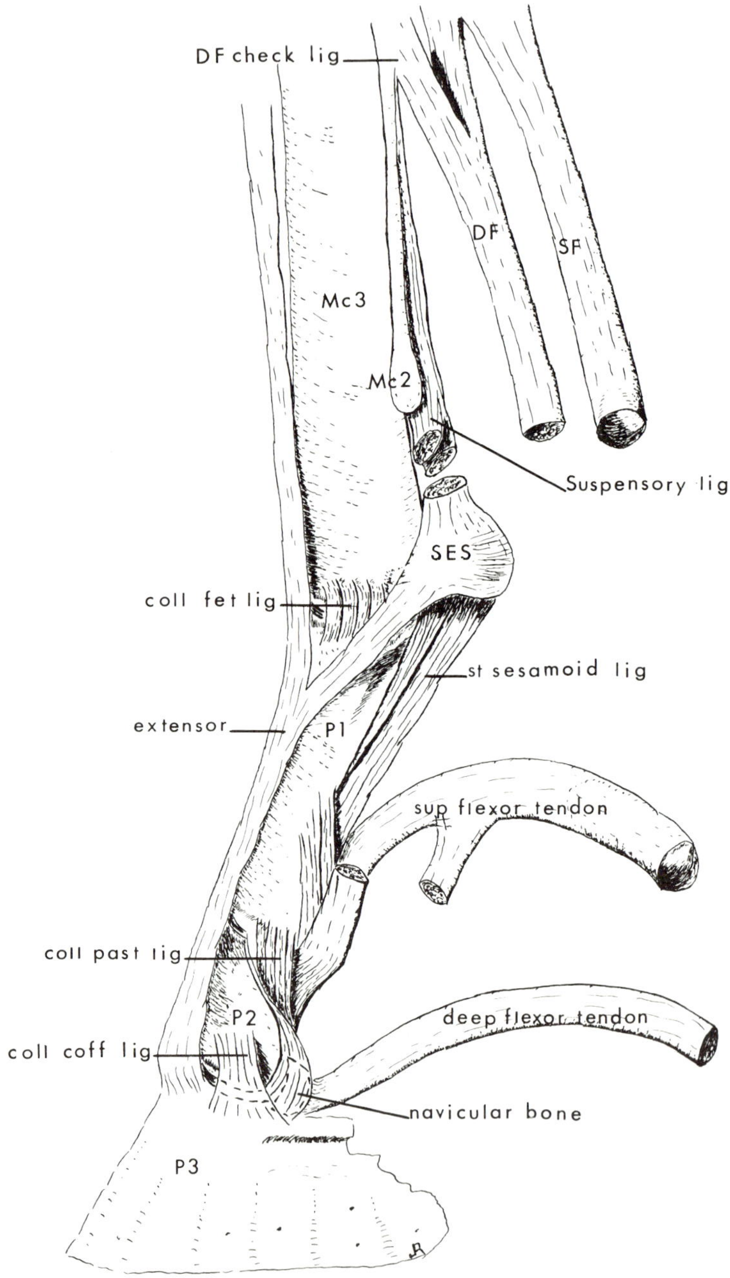

FIG. 29. Medial view of metacarpus and digit. The tendons and suspensory have been transected and the medial insertion of the superficial flexor transected; *lig*, ligament; *coll*, collateral; *coff*, coffin; *past*, pastern; and *SES*, proximal sesamoid bone.

Dissection

Foreleg

Transect the flexor tendons and suspensory ligament just above the proximal sesamoid bones (palpate). Open the digital synovial sheath (72) by sliding the knife down in the sheath and cutting outward through the medial insertion of the superficial flexor tendon (Fig. 29). There is a well developed mesotendon running from the deep face of the deep flexor tendon to the parietal wall of the digital synovial sheath. It is normal. Grasp the deep flexor tendon with a paper towel (it's slippery!). Hold the knife blade flat against the palmar surface of the pastern and, drawing down and out on the DF tendon, cut distad to open first the navicular bursa and second (just in front of the navicular bursa) the proximal palmar extension of the coffin joint. Open both as widely as possible. Holding the hoof firmly with the left hand and pushing down, insert the tip of the knife into the coffin joint and with the knife tip as a fulcrum, always within the joint, lever the knife abaxially, severing the medial collateral ligament of the coffin joint (Fig. 30). *This dissection is relatively easy in the young animal but is more difficult and dangerous in older horses. Be sure the hands and knife are dry (wrap in paper towel) and work carefully.*

Continue around the front of the hoof with the knife, cutting the fascia, the common extensor tendon, and the lateral collateral ligament of the coffin joint. The lateral collateral ligament is severed most readily from inside the coffin joint. Remove the hoof and its contents. Place the hoof on the table and cut around the navicular bone until it can be removed and examined (Fig. 31).

Palpate and slice the cartilages of the third phalanx. Palpate and examine the straight sesamoid ligament.

Pressing down on the distal end of P2, transect the insertion of the straight sesamoid ligament on the complementary fibrocartilage of P2. Transect the medial collateral ligament, opening the pastern joint (Figs. 32, 33). Pressing down on the distal end of P2 tenses the collateral ligament, and the joint is more easily opened. The pastern joint is one of the more difficult to open because of its small size. Multiple parallel slices and maintaining firm pressure on the distal end of P2 much simplifies the task.

Carefully palpate P2 and the distal end of P1 for evidence of the new bone formation of either articular or nonarticular ringbone (84).

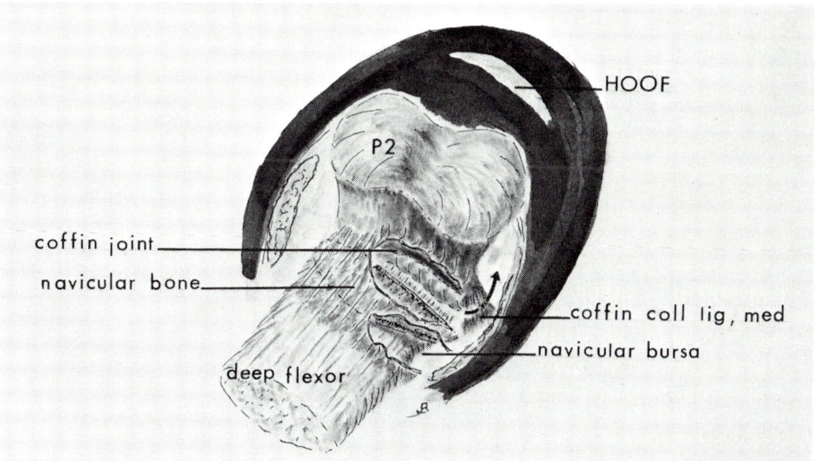

FIG. 30. Opening the navicular bursa and the coffin joint. The *arrow* shows the direction for severing the medial collateral ligament of the coffin joint (*coffin coll lig, med*). P2 would, of course, still be united with P1 at this stage but is shown separated for clarity.

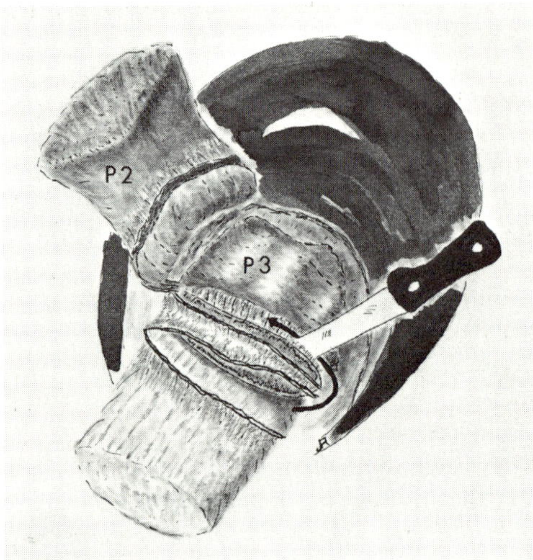

FIG. 31. Medial collateral ligament severed and P2 tipped away. The knife is freeing the navicular bone. In fact, the lateral collateral ligament would also have been severed and the hoof and P3 completely removed from attachments to P2 before removing the navicular bone.

Press down on the distal end of P1 and sever the medial collateral ligament of the fetlock. Pass the tip of the knife proximally between the palmar surface of MC3 and the medial sesamoid bone to the earlier tendon transection and cut out, severing the medial collateral ligament of the sesamoid bone. Open the dorsal synovial pouch on MC3 (Figs. 32 and 34).

Inspect and palpate the branches of the suspensory ligament. Slice the intersesamoidean ligament between the two sesamoid bones. Palpate MC2, MC3, and MC4.

Insert the knife between the suspensory and the flexor tendons and run it proximally to open the carpal synovial sheath, continuing proximally above the carpus to expose the SF check ligament. By blunt and sharp dissection isolate and examine the DF check ligament (Fig. 35).

Pressing down on the distal end of MC3, flex the carpus and transect the medial collateral ligament, opening the radiocarpal joint. Be sure to cut the synovial "flaps" on the dorsal aspect, so that all surfaces can be examined. Open the

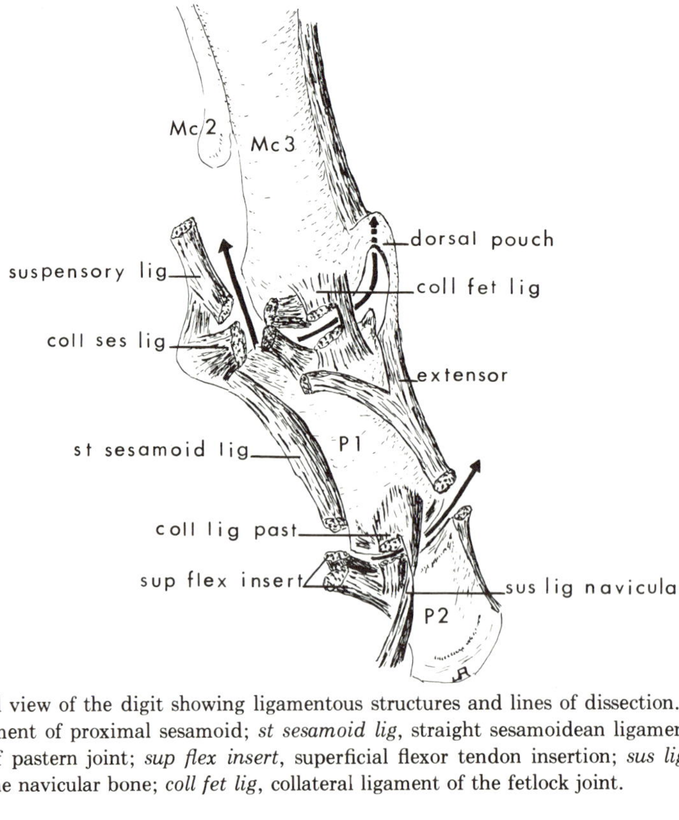

FIG. 32. Medial view of the digit showing ligamentous structures and lines of dissection. Labels are: *coll ses lig*, collateral ligament of proximal sesamoid; *st sesamoid lig*, straight sesamoidean ligament; *coll lig past*, collateral ligament of pastern joint; *sup flex insert*, superficial flexor tendon insertion; *sus lig navicular*, suspensory ligament of the navicular bone; *coll fet lig*, collateral ligament of the fetlock joint.

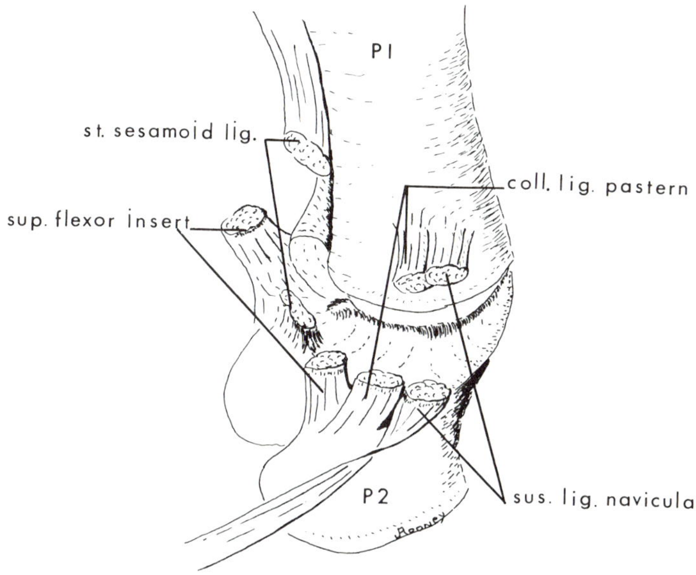

FIG. 33. The pastern joint opened. Figure labels are as for Figure 32.

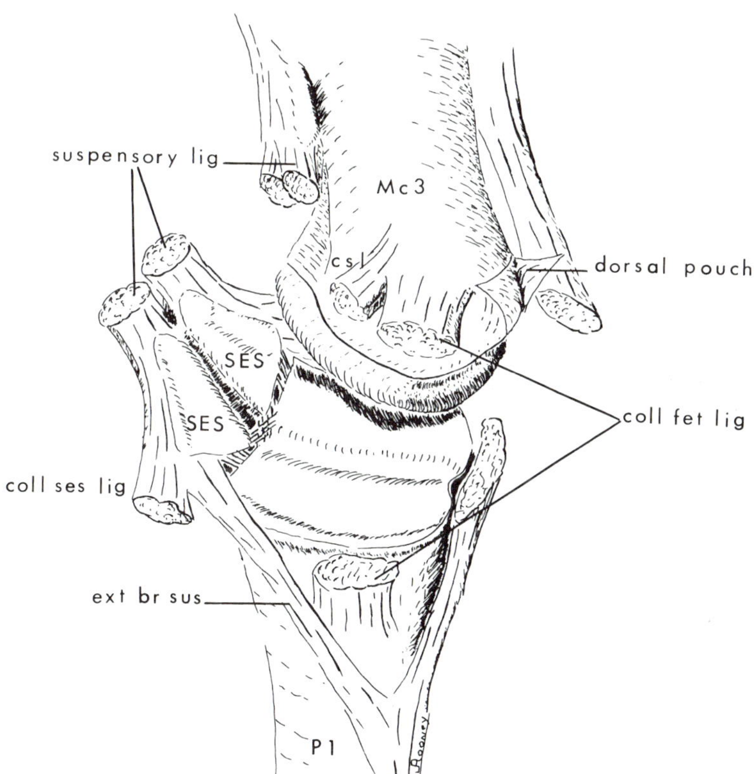

FIG. 34. The fetlock joint opened. Labels are as for Figure 32. *SES*, the proximal sesamoid bones; *csl*, MC3 insertion of the collateral sesamoid ligament; *coll ses lig*, the sesamoid bone insertion; *ext br sus*, extensor branch of the suspensory ligament.

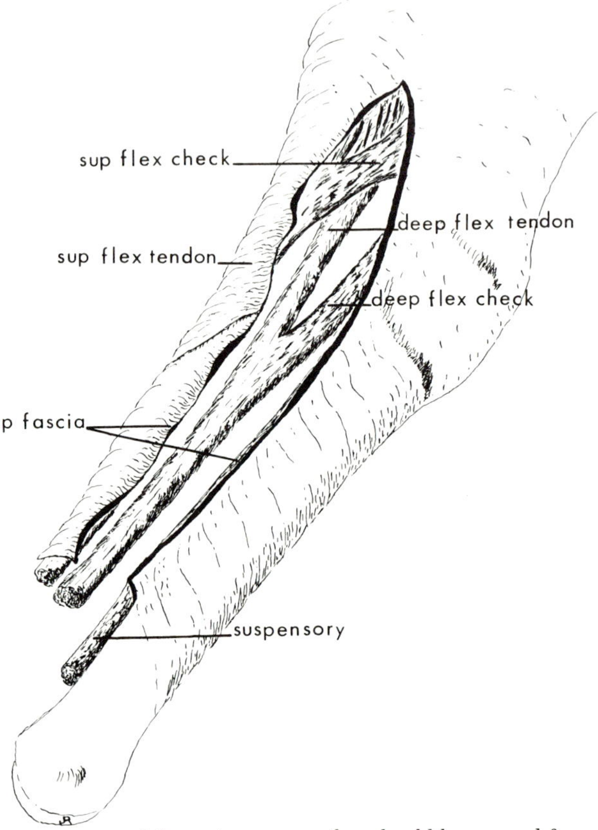

FIG. 35. Tendinous structures of the metacarpus as they should be exposed for examination.

intracarpal joint, reflecting the joint capsule flaps in order to examine all surfaces (Fig. 36).

The adult carpometacarpal joint is difficult to open. After considerable negative experience, I have abandoned opening this joint unless radiographs, palpation, or inspection indicate that lesions are present. Purulent arthritis often occurs in this joint (as well as many others; it is not a preferential site), and the joint should be examined in foals and in older horses with a history of joint infection or lesions elsewhere.

Press down on the distal end of the radius and sever the medial collateral ligament of the elbow, continuing the incision on the dorsal aspect to open the joint widely. Remove the pectoral muscle and palpate the collateral ligament before cutting (Fig. 37).

Pressing down on the proximal end of the radius, open the shoulder joint by transecting the tendon of the subscapularis muscle. If the cut is properly and widely laid, the biceps brachii tendon will be transected also. Open the bicipital bursa widely. Locate and examine the coracobrachialis bursa between the tendon of the muscle and the medial epicondyle of the proximal end of the humerus (Fig. 37).

Thoroughly slice and examine the muscles of the forearm and shoulder.

Rearleg

From the hock down the procedure is the same as described for the foreleg. Be certain to palpate Mt2 and Mt4 on the lateral side for splints. The tarsal synovial sheath is opened in the same manner as the carpal sheath. There is no SF check ligament, the tendon having comparable attachments to the tuber calcis. The DF check ligament is thinner than in the foreleg and may be absent.

The intratarsal and tarsometatarsal joints are

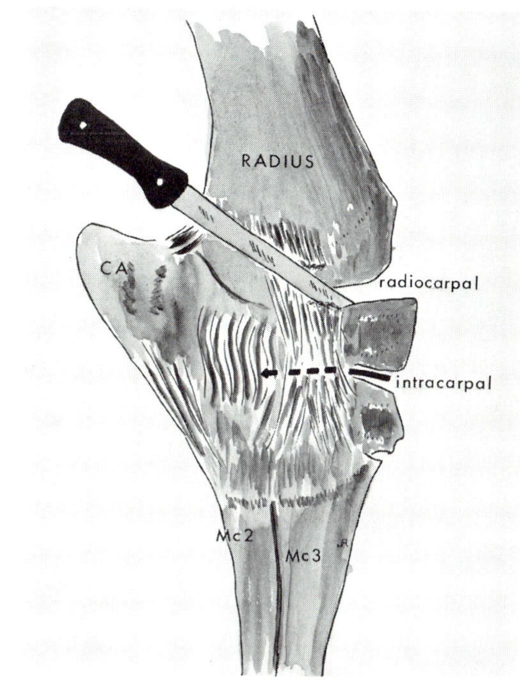

FIG. 36. Opening the carpus. The knife is severing the medial collateral ligament and opening the radiocarpal joint. The *arrow* indicates the line for the second incision into the intracarpal joint.

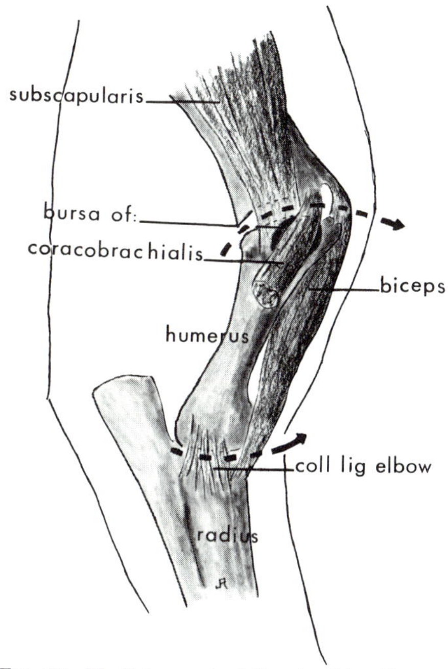

FIG. 37. Medial aspect of the shoulder-elbow area with the dissection lines for each joint indicated. Note the position of the coracobrachialis bursa and that the biceps brachii is transected.

exceedingly difficult to open with the knife. The area should be carefully palpated for the presence of new bone formation. If new bone is present or if there is a history of rearleg lameness, the hock should be removed for radiography, dissection, and/or sawing.

Pressing down on the distal end of MT3, transect the medial collateral ligament of the tarsus and transect the tibialis cranialis and peroneus tertius (Fig. 38), opening the tibiotarsal joint widely. Carefully palpate the plantar tarsal ligament for evidence of thickening (curb).

Press down on the distal end of the tibia; palpate and sever the medial femorotibial collateral ligament, continuing the incision dorsally to the border of the medial patellar ligament. Take care to leave the medial meniscus with the tibia. Direct the tip of the knife proximally along the medial trochlea of the femur parallel to the medial patellar ligament. Cut outward, severing the medial femoropatellar ligament. Transect the quadriceps femoris insertions on the patella and reflect the patella laterally (Fig. 39).

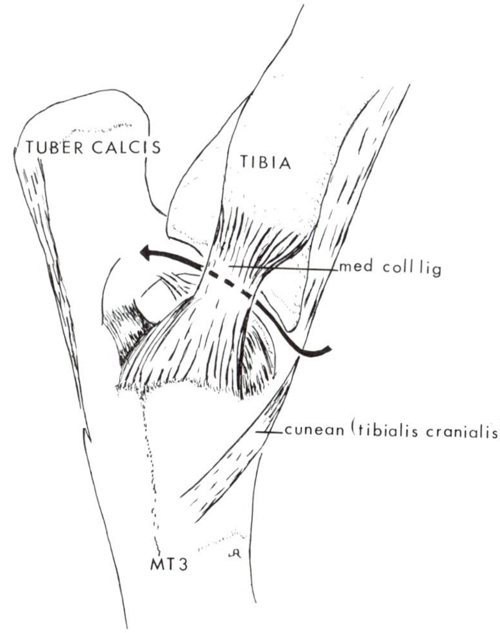

FIG. 38. Opening the tibiotarsal joint.

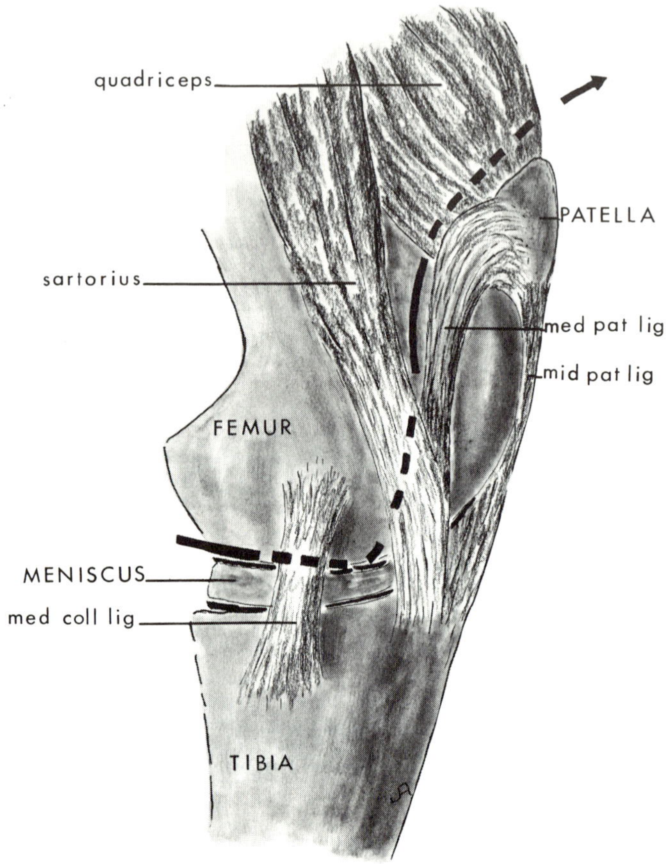

FIG. 39. Medial aspect of stifle with the dissection lines shown. Labels are: *med coll lig*, medial femorotibial collateral ligament; *med* and *mid pat lig*, medial and middle patellar ligaments, respectively.

Insert the knife between the condyles of the femur and stab in to sever the cruciate ligaments (Fig. 40). The joint will drop open, exposing the lateral femorotibial joint. Locate the medial and lateral collateral ligaments and reflect them distad, opening the constant bursa between the medial ligament and the tibia and the inconstant bursa between the lateral ligament and the tibia. Continue reflecting the lateral ligament to its insertion on the head of the fibula. Open the tibiofibular joint. Cut the ligaments of the menisci in order to completely examine both the menisci and the articular surfaces of the tibia.

Open the coxofemoral joint if this has not already been done. The trochanteric bursa may be examined by either removing the leg or rolling the carcass over. Examine the iliopsoas muscle, following it to its insertion on the minor trochanter of the femur. Slice and examine the muscles of the thigh. Carefully palpate and slice the biceps, semitendinosus, and semimembranosus muscles particularly in the area of fibrosing myopathy (distal semitendinosus).

Interpretation

It is impossible, within the present context, to consider all possible lesions of the locomotor system. The present material, together with that presented earlier (84), covers at least some portion of the field.

Frequently there is a shallow, narrow groove on the palmar face of the navicular bone. It is normal and may serve as a

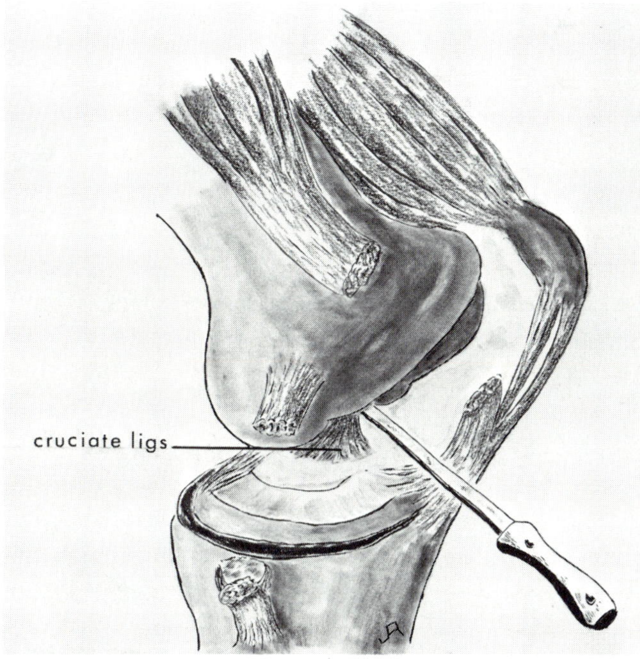

FIG. 40. Completing the dissection of the stifle. The knife is severing the cruciate ligaments. Note the bursa under the severed medial femorotibial collateral ligament.

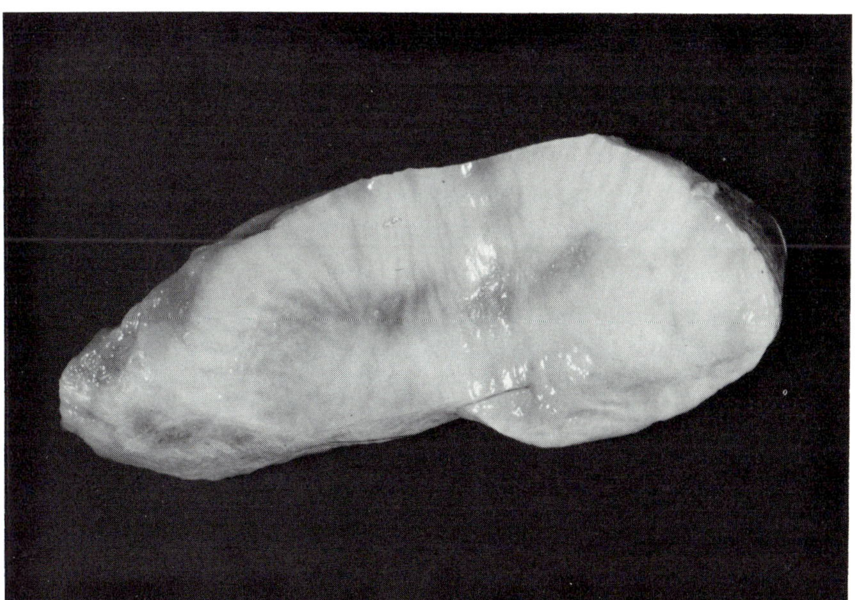

FIG. 41. Transverse groove (darker) on the palmar face of the navicular bone. This is an inconstant but normal finding.

synovial fossa (Fig. 41). Lesions of the navicular area are of two basic types. The common navicular disease begins as an acute bursitis with yellowing, fraying, and erosion of the deep face of the DF tendon and the articular fibrocartilage of the navicular bone (Fig. 42). Many older horses show such yellowish discoloration to some degree and clinically significant navicular disease cannot be diagnosed on this basis alone. Even quite marked bursal, tendon, cartilage, and bony charges can be present without clinical evidence of navicular lameness. The clinical history, results of nerve blocks, bursal injections, and both antemortem and postmortem radiographs should be carefully evaluated. The same amount of damage in an old broodmare may be of considerably less clinical significance than in a four-year-old hunter.

The literature abounds with work purporting to show that osteitis or osteosis of the navicular bone is the primary lesion. I believe that the bone changes are secondary to damage to the articular fibrocartilage—the bone fibrosis, "cyst" formation, and osteophytosis following the usual pattern of arthrosis in any joint. Since the cartilage is fibrocartilage, marked changes can occur without the obvious gross changes so familiar in hyaline articular cartilage. If the specimen is allowed to dry in the air for a short time, the erosive lesions in fibrocartilage will become more apparent. Also, fibrocartilage appears to have a greater capacity for healing than hyaline cartilage. Erosive lesions may occur and subchondral bone changes may develop, followed by healing of the fibrocartilage. Both radiologically and at autopsy, then, the subchondral bone changes may appear to be primary.

Osteolysis, radiographic widening of the vascular markings of the navicular bone, is often considered characteristic of navic-

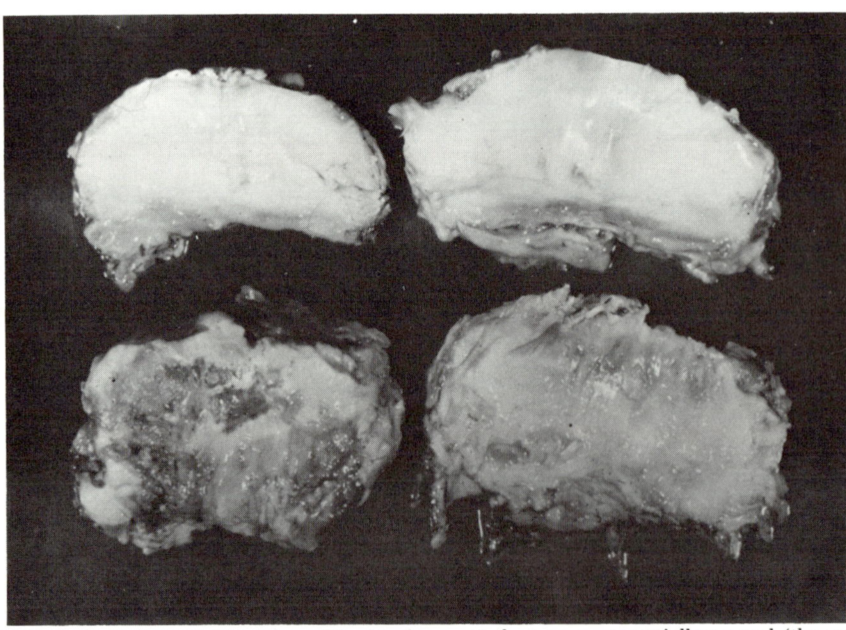

FIG. 42. Navicular lesions, palmar view. The two bones at the top are essentially normal (the apparent defects are knife artefacts). The two bottom bones show severe erosion and destruction of the fibrocartilage.

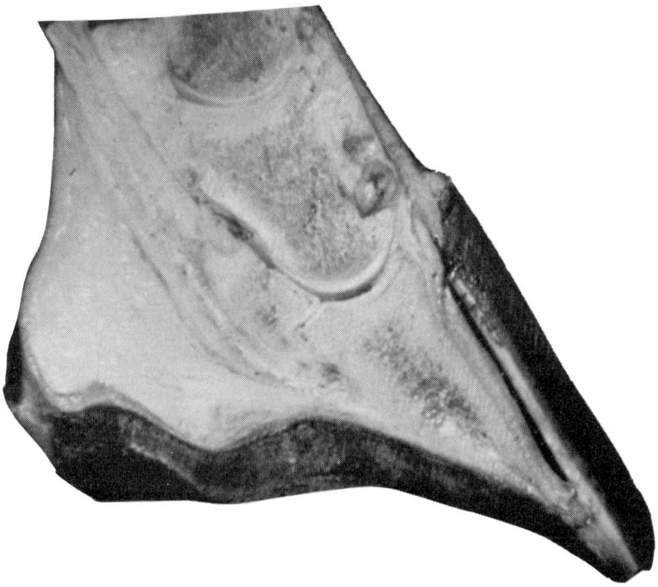

FIG. 43. Acute laminitis of short duration. There has been separation of the hoof from P3 and the space is filled with free blood, which appears as the dark line to the left of the white laminar horn.

ular disease. This is true *only* if the widening is demonstrated on serial radiographs of the same bone of the same horse.

The second type of navicular lesion is a spur of new bone formation at either or both ends of the navicular bone, sometimes accompanied by new bone formation along the distal border of the navicular bone (insertion of distal coffin-navicular ligament). There are no lesions of the cartilage-tendon surfaces. The causes of both these lesions have been considered in detail elsewhere (84).

Although the etiology of laminitis remains obscure, there are several points which may be recorded (see Chapter 8), (57, 71). Recent work has shown that horses fed a special diet will frequently, if not routinely, develop acute laminitis (97). Arteriography has shown, that in these animals, there is marked vasoconstriction of the digital arterial system as the laminitis develops (15). My own limited histological studies of cases of acute laminitis of less than one week's duration as well as certain of Obel's (71) pictures suggest that there is a vacuolar degeneration of the laminar epidermis, a lesion consistent with acute ischemia. The toxic material or materials, then, may be acting as vasoconstrictors of small dermal arteries with resultant ischemic necrosis of the laminar epidermis. The obvious mechanical predilection of the hoof and, particularly, the forehoof results in the classical clinical and pathological changes once necrosis has occurred. Vasodilation routinely follows a period of vasospasm, resulting in the classical picture of blood "pooling" in the hoof (Fig. 43). This outline is consistent with but not identical to that of Obel (71).

Pony laminitis is most often of subacute type (Hickman's classification) (40), occurring in fat ponies on pasture. In such ponies pathological examination rarely shows the clear separation of the horny and sensitive laminae, so obvious in horses, no matter how severe or chronic the clinical signs of lameness. Careful examination reveals only tearing away of the distal, dorsal "tip" of P3 from the hoof wall with, in acute cases, hemorrhage in the area (Fig. 44).

I suggest, therefore, that most pony laminitis is not of the classical type seen in horses. Perhaps it is more correct to state that there appear to be two types of laminitis in the horse. The classical type is caused by unknown toxic materials which cause vasoconstriction of the dermal arteries, ischemic epidermal necrosis, and sensitive-insensitive laminae separation because of the necrosis and the mechanics of the single digit. The pony type (most common in fat ponies but perhaps seen in fat or badly hoof-trimmed horses, also) appears to be a mechanical tearing away of sensitive-insensitive laminae at the apex of the coffin bone. This concept has also been alluded to by Obel (71). This type of mechanical laminitis is predisposed to by: (1) obesity and (2) long toe. The mechanics are summarized in Figure 45. The long toe increases the moment arm around the tip of the coffin bone, increasing the force and thereby tearing the sensitive-insensitive junction. Increasing the mass of the animal (obesity) will enhance this tearing tendency because of greater resistance to the breaking over of the hoof at the end of the stride.

The bilateral nature of classical laminitis is obvious. In the pony type the bilateral nature can be explained, in part at least, by the acute, severe pain in one foot which promptly causes the animal to carry more load on the opposite leg and tear that foot quickly after the first. The therapy for pony laminitis is obvious: shorten and round the toe and place the pony on a radical diet. (The latter is difficult.)

One further point may be made. So-called road founder could be of either type. Exhaustion leads to ileus and toxic product formation (alimentary laminitis). On the other hand a long-toed animal sub-

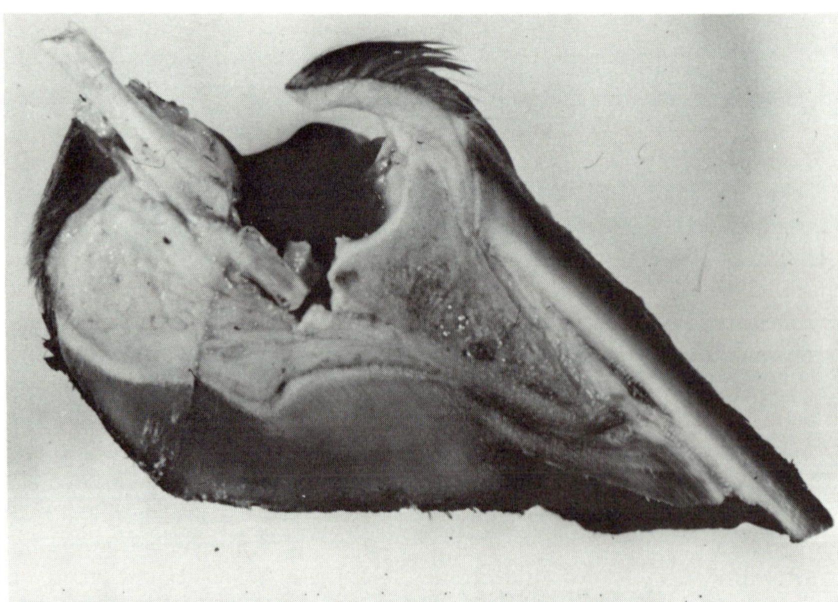

FIG. 44. Acute pony laminitis. Note the small area of dehiscence and hemorrhage near apex of P3.

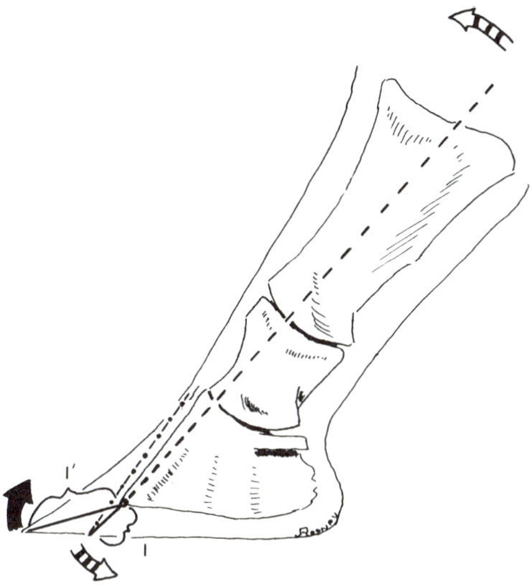

FIG. 45. Suggested mechanics of pony-type laminitis. With a long toe the moment arm l' is greater than l and more force will be applied near the apex of the coffin bone. The *upper striped arrow* indicates the movement of the digit toward the end of the stride, breaking over. The coffin bone moves in the direction of *lower striped arrow*. The resistance, exerting force at the apex of the coffin, is indicated by the *solid arrow* and will be greater in the animal with a long toe. -·-·-, indicates the position of a proper, normal hoof wall with moment arm l around apex of coffin bone.

jected to prolonged work might tear at the toe in the pony laminitis fashion. It should be obvious, perhaps, that corns or bruising of the sole could produce acute lameness difficult to distinguish from road founder.

Sidebone is quite uncommon as a clinical problem in the modern light horse breeds. Usually the ossification begins at the junction of the cartilage with the wing of the coffin bone, but separate ossification centers may be seen. The clinical significance of relatively minor degrees of ossification needs to be carefully evaluated in terms of the previous history of the animal.

Pedal osteitis or osteosis is becoming a popular clinical diagnosis. Since the coffin bone can be examined only with difficulty at autopsy, I am unable to offer any meaningful opinion. Routine postmortem radiography is needed.

Ringbone may be either articular or nonarticular (84). In the former, there is erosion of the pastern joint cartilage on the dorsomedial aspect of the joint with the subsequent development of osteophytes. With nonarticular ringbone, new bone formation is usually restricted to ligamentous insertions around the pastern joint. Articular ringbone, although uncommon, at best, seems to be somewhat more frequent in the lighter, racing breeds whereas nonarticular ringbone is more common in the coarser breeds or coarser individuals of the light breeds. In the coarser horse, with advancing age slight new bone formation may become apparent at ligamentous insertions. Such "excrescences" may be barely apparent radiographically and should be carefully evaluated before being considered the cause of clinical lameness.

At this point it may be well to emphasize the advantages of postmortem radiography. If osteophytes are palpable or suspected, a radiograph may be taken to confirm the suspicion and to provide assistance in determining what to do next. Sharp dissection does not clearly demonstrate nonarticular lesions of the pastern, and radiographs and palpation must be used to determine whether maceration will be used to fully expose the bone changes, sections taken for histology, or careful dissection undertaken to retain continuity of bone-soft tissue relationships. Only in the latter, a most tedious case, can sectioning and/or maceration follow the initial procedure. In the absence of radiographs it must be the procedure of choice.

I shall digress here to consider old age changes in the articular cartilage of any and all joints. With age the normally bluish-white articular cartilage fades to a tan-yellow. Young cartilage is resilient and thick, becoming thinner and firmer with age. Small erosions scattered at random over the joint surface, rarely penetrating to the underlying bone, frequently appear in this old, fragile cartilage. So far as I know these "wearings" of old cartilage are not associated with clinical lameness. Subchondral cysts and pits and "dimpling" of the articular cartilage have been considered elsewhere (84).

Pathological changes are common in the fetlock. Arthrosis occurs on the dorsal lip of the articular surface of P1 and the corresponding dorsal aspect of MC3, the area uncovered by opening the dorsal synovial pouch. The normal synovial fringe in this area is destroyed if the lesions are sufficiently severe. With sufficient damage in this area there will be clinically apparent acute or chronic swelling (fibrosis) known as osselets. Pathological fractures, so-called chips, may occur through the arthrotic areas on P1. There may also be wearing, arthrosis, and fraying of the articular cartilage along the line of demarcation between the sesamoid and P1 articular surfaces of the distal end of MC3 (84). This may be accompanied by new bone formation along the basal borders of the sesamoid bones. Wear lines are common, usually but not invariably accompanying the above mentioned lesions. Small translucent dark patches may be present in the intersesamoidian ligament. They appear to be chondroid tissue, and I believe (but see (7)) they are of no clinical significance.

The periosteal proliferation which accompanies bucked shin is readily palpable on the dorsal aspect of MC3.

Bowed tendon is easily recognized, and the careful prosector will become convinced that the primary damage is always in the SF tendon. In my experience damage to the DF tendon has been limited to the check ligament. It may be worth noting at this point that in cases of tendoligamentous tearing, except ones of very long standing, there will be evidence of fibrosis, fresh granulation tissue, and bleeding in the same tendon. It is reasonable that once tearing occurs and granulation and fibrosis develop the tearing process may be repeated. That is, the new young granulation tissue is not properly oriented for tensile strain and is subject to retearing every time the coffin and fetlock joints move.

The lateral aspect of the articular surface of the distal end of the radius is a common site for traumatic arthrosis, but there is rarely a mirror lesion on the intermediate carpal bone. The opposing surfaces of the radial carpal bone and C3 are also a common site for severe arthrosis. In older horses one frequently finds these arthrotic changes in what may be considered a burned-out state. That is, the damage occurred years before and only the inactive results remain. The burned-out lesion is characterized by a lack of hyperemia and smooth edges, apparently as a result of incomplete healing of the articular cartilage. More active lesions, with their ragged edges and hyperemic surroundings, may have strands of pannus-like tissue extending from the synovial membrane to and over the lesions. This pannus formation is particularly striking in joints which have been surgically curetted.

The prosector should note the white line which demarcates the lateral epicondyle of the distal end of the radius. This portion of the articular surface is derived from the distal end of the ulna and remains demarcated throughout life in most horses.

The synovial fossae on the distal end of the humerus, proximal end of the radius, and the olecranon process of the ulna are quite variable in size. They are not present at birth and appear to develop during the third and fourth postnatal month. They may be very small and barely perceptible or quite large and striking. No pathological significance should be attached to them, no matter what the size. Wear lines occur commonly in the elbow and suggest that the animal has been lame at some time, either in the same or some other leg. If wear lines are found in both elbows, ataxia may have been present during life and should be kept in mind when the central nervous system is examined. The wear lines probably do not cause clinical signs of lameness.

The central portion of the glenoid fossa of the scapula always has an irregular, folded appearance after the third to fourth month of life. The nature of this area is not completely clear, but it is definitely normal and quite variable in size and distinctness. It probably serves as a synovial fossa. The head of the humerus flattens toward the lateral aspect, and a rather distinct groove may be present. This groove also probably serves as a synovial fossa.

Synovial fossae routinely occur in the tibiotarsal joint on both the distal end of the tibia and the tibiotarsal bone. They vary enormously in size. An area of osteochondrosis dissecans is occasionally present at the dorsal end of the intermediate ridge of the distal end of the tibia. This lesion, a distinct piece of bone surrounded by cartilage, is always bilateral and never associated with clinical signs of lameness in my experience. It should not be considered a fracture.

The stifle joint is remarkably free of lesions. Purulent arthritis and its aftermath, articular pits, foldings, mounds, and subchondral masses of fibrous tissue (so-called subchondral cysts), are common, however. Rupture of the cruciate ligaments is very rare, usually avulses bone, and is clinically strikingly disabling.

The hip joint is also rarely the site of clinically significant lesions. In a case of stringhalt, the course of the obturator nerve should be carefully traced (84).

Sacroiliac luxation occurs in horses and is easily discerned in the live animal. The entire lumbosacral area should be removed and the sacroiliac areas carefully fleshed out in order to demonstrate the lesions (78, 84).

Often it will be desirable to split one or more long bones with the band saw in order to examine bone marrow. Most of the marrow in mature horses, with the exception of ribs, sternum, and vertebrae, is fatty. With cachexia this fatty marrow undergoes serous atrophy. It should be noted that large islands of red marrow are normally present in the humerus and, especially, the femur (16). Their presence does not indicate equine infectious anemia.

Foals with pyemia (joint-ill, navel-ill) may have varying degrees of acute synovitis. The proximal limb joints are somewhat more frequently affected than the distal joints. There will be severe hyperemia of the synovial membrane and dirty brownish, yellow discoloration of the synovial fluid (Fig. 46). Strands and masses of fibrin and purulent material may be present. Shigella infection never causes articular cartilage damage, whereas streptococcal infections regularly cause erosions, scattered at random over the joint surface. Total joint destruction is most often associated with persistent streptococcal infections (Fig. 47).

Polyarthritis, a poorly understood condition, has been seen sporadically in young

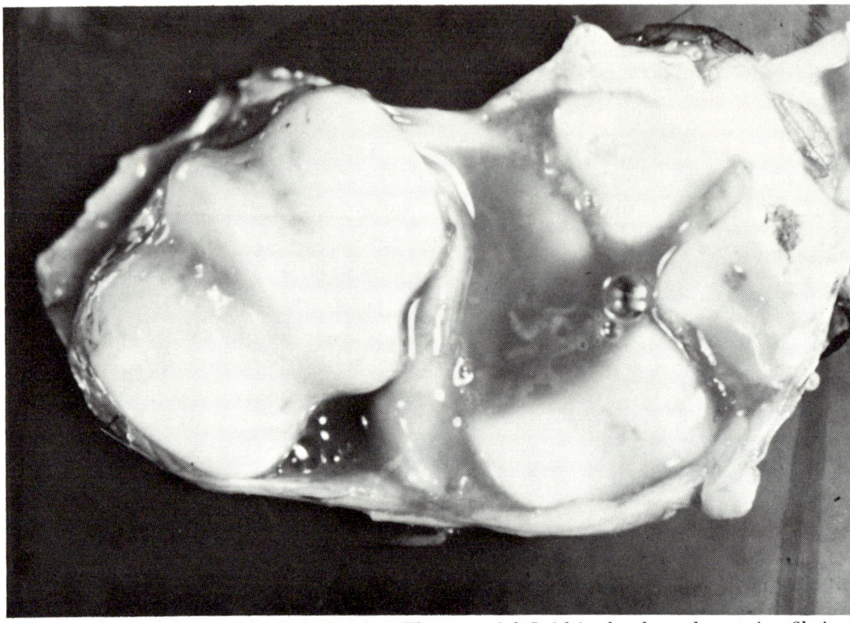

FIG. 46. Acute bacterial synovitis, fetlock joint. The synovial fluid is cloudy and contains fibrin flakes.

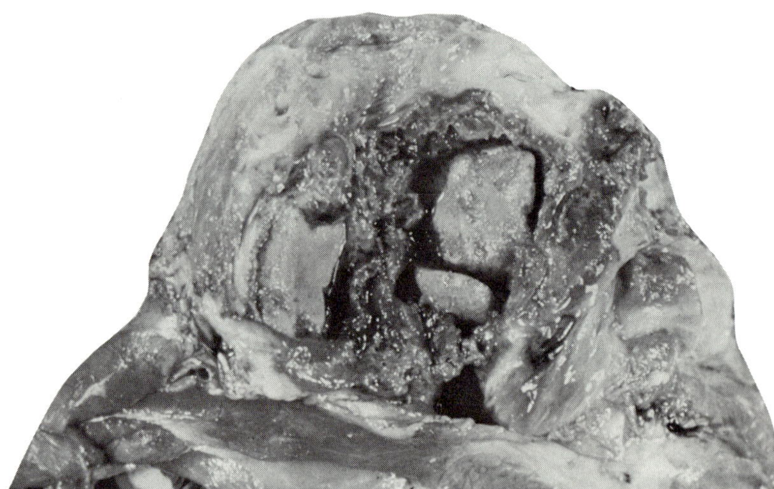

FIG. 47. Shoulder joint totally destroyed by bacterial infection. The remnants of the glenoid of the scapula are to the left and the head of the humerus to the right.

foals. The animal is acutely and severely lame as a result of flaking off of large parts of the articular cartilages, particularly of the more distal limb joints. If the animal is allowed to live, these erosions heal over by one year of age, with irregular mounds and folds of hyaline cartilage. Pathologically, the process is an osteochrondrosis, but the cause is not known.

Dirty discoloration and frank hemorrhage into the synovial fluid is common in horses that have thrashed about before death, as with colic, for example.

Azoturia is not uncommon in horses and

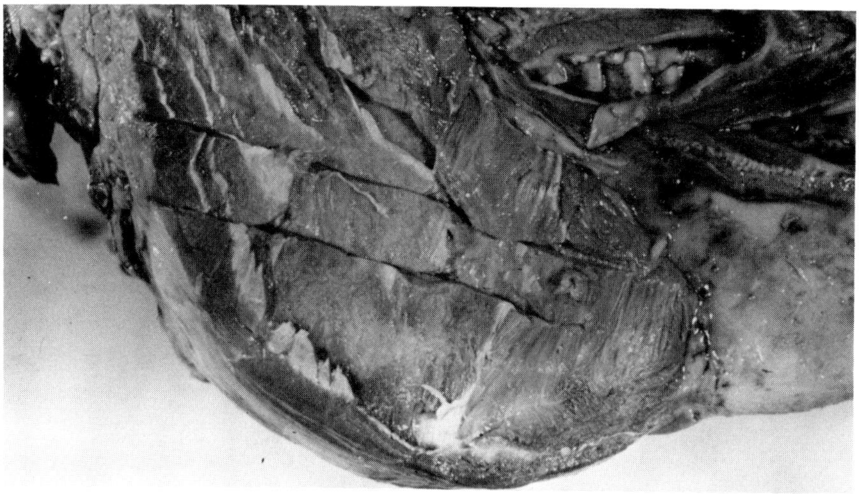

FIG. 48. Maxillary myopathy. Normal muscle near ventral border of mandible, then, white tags of tendinous inscriptions and, in the center, the pale tan degenerated muscle tissue.

presents as a striking clinical and pathological entity (88). Tying-up is apparently similar to azoturia, but the pathology of the latter condition has not been described. I quote from Jubb and Kennedy (50): "Paralytic myoglobinuria typically occurs very shortly after beginning exercise following some days of rest on full working rations. Profound weakness of the hind limbs occurs suddenly, so that the animal becomes unable to move, and this is accompanied by sweating and generalized tremors. The affected muscles, which are typically those of the gluteal, femoral, and lumbar groups, are swollen and board-like in their rigidity; their dissolution begins soon after the onset and myoglobin is passed in the urine, which is thereby discoloured to dark brown. Severely affected horses become recumbent, a symptom which is often a prelude to death from myoglobinuric nephrosis or intercurrent decubital infection. Such is the usual theme, but there are variations in the severity, course, and the nature of exercise which is always necessary to precipitate the disease.

The morbid, gross changes in muscle are most consistent and evident in the dorsal and ventral lumbar masses, the gluteals and the quadriceps groups, but the actual distribution of changes is more widespread than is evident grossly. The affected muscles may show little gross change other than moderate swelling and distinct pallor with an increased amount of interstitial fluid. Other muscles, or portions of them, exhibit changes in patches or streaks in which the tissue is grayish-yellow and friable and in some cases beset with small fusiform or linear hemorrhages. . . .

The kidneys are slightly swollen but of normal contour. The cut surface of the cortex is discoloured brownish and that of the medulla shows deep red-brown radial streaks."

Nutritional myopathy has been described in horses (24, 50). I have seen only one case, a nine-year-old Shetland pony mare. The maxillary and temporal muscles were involved (so-called maxillary myositis) (Fig. 48).

FIVE

The Head and Spinal Column

Dissection

Examine the eyes, reflect the skin from the lateral surfaces of the head, and slice and examine the parotid and mandibular salivary glands and parotid lymph nodes. Slice and examine the masseter muscles. A good gross examination of the eye is difficult. If there are gross changes or clinically relevant history, the eyes should be removed and fixed for dissection and sectioning. Dissection of the fresh eye is useless and only destroys the specimen (12, 47).

If the history suggests a brain lesion, remove the calvarium by careful elevation with a chisel after placing saw cuts, as indicated in Figure 49. Incise the dura and tip the head backward, tipping the brain out of the cranial cavity and severing the cranial nerves and stalk of the pituitary. Remove the pituitary by incising the thick dura mater over the sella turcica and freeing the gland from the plexus of surrounding vessels. By carefully freeing the dura from the floor of the cranial cavity, the pituitary can be brought out with the brain and with the stalk intact.

Remove the incisor teeth by a transverse saw cut behind the bodies of the premaxilla and mandible. Saw the head in half on the midline. Examine the nasal passages, turbinate bones, ethmoids, frontal sinuses, and guttural pouches. Remove the nasal septum, which will usually be on one-half of the head.

Make frontal saw cuts through each half of the head to open the maxillary sinuses. Note that all saw cuts should be placed to avoid the teeth.

Routinely, when no brain lesions are suspected, simply remove the incisors as described and split the head on the midline, removing and examining the two halves of the brain.

The spinal cord presents tedious, if not difficult, technical problems. Remove the entire back bone, remove the muscle, and palpate and search carefully for evidence of abnormalities. Saw or disarticulate the back into convenient segments: cervical, upper thoracic, lower thoracic, lumbosacral. If possible, postmortem radiographs should be taken, particularly if malformations or masses of new bone are apparent.

When ataxia is the presenting clinical sign, I feel it is mandatory to disarticulate the cervical portion of the vertebral column in order to search for the malformations of "wobbler." The remainder of the vertebral column may be sawed just lateral to the spinal cord, barely opening the spinal canal, and the cord removed intact for examination.

Cervical nerves 1 and 2 (atlas and axis) are first severed with scissors or a long, thin-bladed knife within the spinal canal. C2 and C3 are then disarticulated. From the dorsal surface both intervertebral articulations are opened and the ligamenta flava is opened, exposing the spinal cord within the dura. The specimen is turned over and the intervertebral disk located by flexing the specimen. Cut down to the disk and insert the knife tip into the disk as deeply as possible. Cut abaxially in both directions. Continue the cut through the muscles to join the cuts in the joint capsules of the intervertebral articulations. Try to disarticulate by flexing C2 and C3 over the table edge. If severe resistance is encountered,

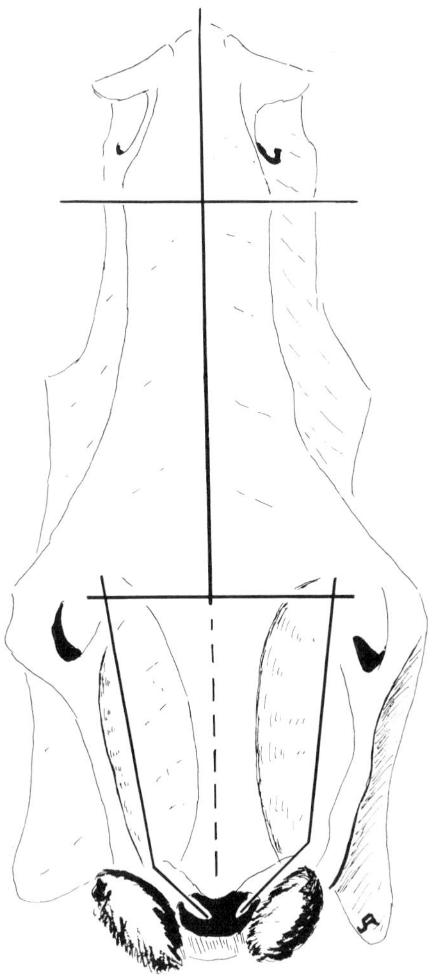

FIG. 49. Dorsal view of skull with position of saw cuts for removing the brain intact and/or for splitting the skull after removal of the incisors.

repeat the cuts already described, being certain that no strips of ligamentous tissue remain. Carefully cut the intervertebral disk closer to the dorsal part of the annulus fibrosus, avoiding nicking the ventral surface of the spinal cord. Eventually, C1 and C2 will separate as a unit, slipping off the cord because the nerve roots have been severed.

Cut the nerve roots of articulation of C2–3 and proceed to disarticulate C3–4, C4–5, etc. In this manner the cervical cord, within the dura mater, is intact and may be examined in the light of the changes in the intervertebral articulations (84).

Interpretation

The teeth, hard palate, etc., should be carefully examined. I have never seen lesions of the salivary glands. The parotid lymph nodes may have melanotic changes in old gray horses, with or without perineal melanosis.

The dorsomedial part of the guttural pouch should be examined with particular care for the presence of the plaque of gray-green, tough, necrotic debris characteristic of guttural pouch mycosis (Fig. 50) (18). This lesion closely involves the internal carotid artery and glossopharyngeal and vagus nerves. Massive or moderate bleeding may occur as the fungal hyphae (usually *Aspergillus* spp.) in the necrotic plaque invade the internal carotid artery. Pharyngeal paralysis with persistent regurgitation of solid food occurs when nerves are involved by the lesion.

Fungal infections may be encountered also in the sinuses and ethmoid turbinates. These appear to be secondary to either viral or bacterial upper respiratory infection. I have never seen a case of glanders (16).

Strangles (*Streptococcus equi*) is an acute bacterial infection of the nasal mucosa which quickly invades the regional lymph nodes: mandibular and retropharyngeal. Creamy, purulent abscesses are formed which have thick, fibrous walls and frequently rupture to the outside. Occasionally the infection may spread to other lymph nodes, particularly the caudal cervical nodes in the thoracic inlet ("bastard strangles"). Abscessation in this latter area may be unsuspected and cause sudden asphyxial death in young horses.

Rarely in my experience does the purulent process involve one or both guttural pouches. The empyema can persist for

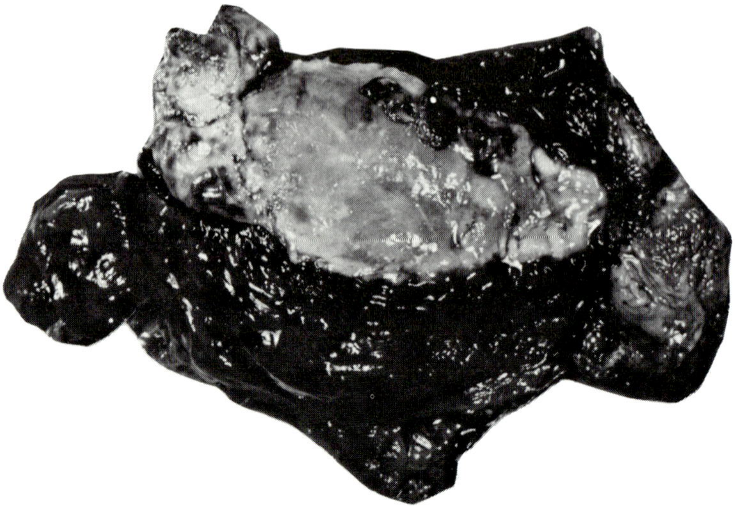

FIG. 50. Guttural pouch mycosis. The mucosa of the pouch is intensely hyperemic (dark) around the plaque of necrotic material (light).

long periods, often asymptomatic, and eventually become inspissated, leaving masses of firm, round balls of caseopurulent material.

Purpura hemorrhagica (51) shall be discussed here since it is so frequently a sequela of strangles infection. I cannot improve upon the description by Jubb and Kennedy (50):

"The equine disease varies from a mild transient reaction to a severe and fatal form. The course may be up to two weeks and relapses may occur. The disease begins with fever and haemorrhages on the nasal mucosa, and these are followed very soon by oedematous swellings. The oedematous swellings may develop as urticarial-like plaques on any part of the body but more frequently the swelling involves the nose, face, and eyelids, and the limbs. The limbs may be swollen to two or three times their normal size. Typically the swellings are cold, painless, pit on pressure, and have a sharp upper margin. Oozing of serum and superficial necrosis may develop in two or three days. Swelling of the head leads to obstruction of the respiratory passages and asphyxia. Viscera, particularly the intestine, may be involved and this causes severe abdominal distress.

"Postmortem examination adds little to what may be deduced from clinical examination. Haemorrhages, even on mucous membranes, may be sparse, and thus the oedematous transudations are the most significant change. The oedema fluid collects in the subcutaneous tissues and the intermuscular fascia, as well as in the abdominal cavity. Lesions in skeletal muscles are rather common, focal, and widespread. The focal lesions may have the greyish colour of degeneration, or be dark red in colour in consequence of local haemorrhage. . . . Patchy or diffuse oedema of the respiratory and alimentary canals occurs, and there may be haemorrhages beneath the serous membranes and the capsules of the kidney and liver.

"Equine purpura haemorrhagica is not associated with a thrombocytopenia or with defects in the coagulation mechanism. There is a progressive or fluctuating anaemia of undetermined pathogenesis, neutrophilia, and eosinopaenia."

Fresh or healed fractures of the great cornu of the hyoid bone may be encountered. There will be hemorrhage in and around the guttural pouch with fresh fractures. Such fractures appear to be of little clinical significance. They may be encountered following destruction if the head strikes the ground heavily or in animals that have been down and thrashing before death.

The nasal septum is apparently a site of predilection for the development of the lesions of the several types of viral upper respiratory infection. Gross lesions are rare, however; fine petechiation is the only gross change, and at that is infrequent. The nasal septum should always be submitted for histological examination in suspected cases of upper respiratory disease.

Nasal amyloidosis has been described (16) as a localized process (not associated with systemic amyloidosis) in the rostral part of the vestibule, nasal septum, and turbinates. I have not seen an example.

Rhinosporidiosis has also been described in the nasal cavity of horses (50), but again I have not personally seen a case.

The frontal and maxillary sinuses are singularly free of pathological changes. They may be involved by any viral or bacterial infection of the upper respiratory system but are rarely involved alone. Maxillary sinus carcinoma (16) does occur and may invade extensively the surrounding bony structures, the orbit, and (rarely) the brain. An occasional maxillary sinus mass, grossly identical to carcinoma, is caused by pigmented, maduromycotic-type fungi.

The intermediate lobe of the pituitary is frequently cystic and/or hyperplastic especially in older horses. The hyperplasia may be so extensive that the term adenoma is applicable (9). I have not seen clinical signs referable to such intermediate lobe hyperplasia-adenoma unless the adenoma pressed upon the hypothalamus (Fig. 51). In such a case the animal will be exceedingly obese, barren, and may fail to shed the long winter haircoat. Frank genital hypoplasia is not appreciable but, in mares at least, the genital tract is inactive.

The brain may be fixed *en toto* or sliced in coronal sections, 2 to 3 mm. thick, with

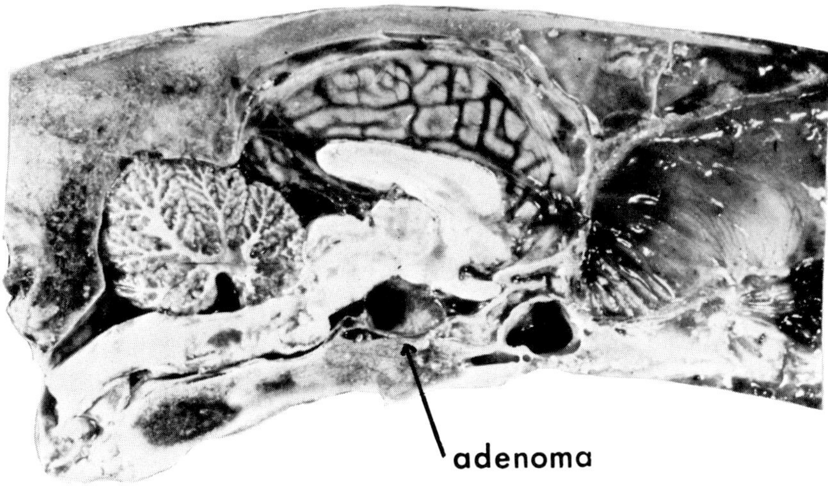

FIG. 51. Adenoma-hyperplasia of the intermediate lobe of the pituitary gland pressing against the hypothalamus.

a sharp, wet knife. The blood vessels on the surface of the brain show virtually all degrees of complexity or hyperemia without pathological significance. Only frank hemorrhages or petechiae should be considered significant. In older animals small accumulations of sand-like material are occasionally present in the choroid plexus of the third ventricle. Large cholesteatomas are rare in the light horse breeds, in my experience.

Horses by their nature are somewhat more prone to traumatic lesions of the skull and brain than other animals. Whenever a contusion is apparent, the prosector should search for both *coup* and *contrecoup* hemorrhages. Most commonly the blow is over the frontal bones and the contrecoup hemorrhage will surround and involve the medulla oblongata. A rather frequent lesion results when a horse rears and strikes an overhead obstacle or falls over backward. The entire occipital-parietal area of the skull may be broken loose from the remainder of the skull with massive hematoma formation. Amazingly, these animals may live for some hours.

Following a fall an animal may be comatose or conscious but unable to rise. While a variety of lesions are seen, fracture of the basisphenoid bone may be most common. This fracture occurs alone or accompanies the other fractures described above, often involving the epiphyseal plate. In some cases the fracture extends to the ear on one or both sides with bleeding into the middle, inner and/or external ear chambers.

Middle ear infections, with startling clinical ataxia, have been observed, but there has been no opportunity for autopsy examination.

Massive hemorrhagic encephalitis occurs occasionally in foals with bacterial pyemia. If one encounters massive hemorrhage in the brain, septic embolization as the cause of hemorrhage should be suspected. Histological studies will be decisive.

Purulent meningitis is occasionally seen in young foals with pyemia.

If the animal was destroyed by shooting, the bullet track through the brain and basisphenoid bone will be apparent. The

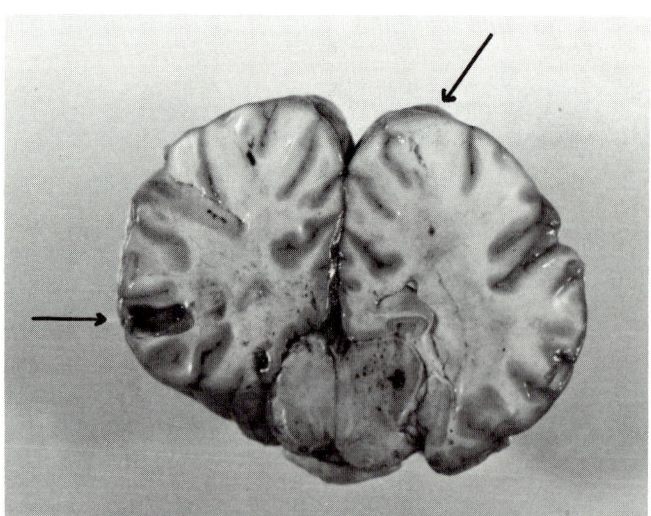

FIG. 52. Moldy corn poisoning. Frank areas of malacia are apparent (*arrows*). There are also numerous hemorrhages in the white matter and corpora.

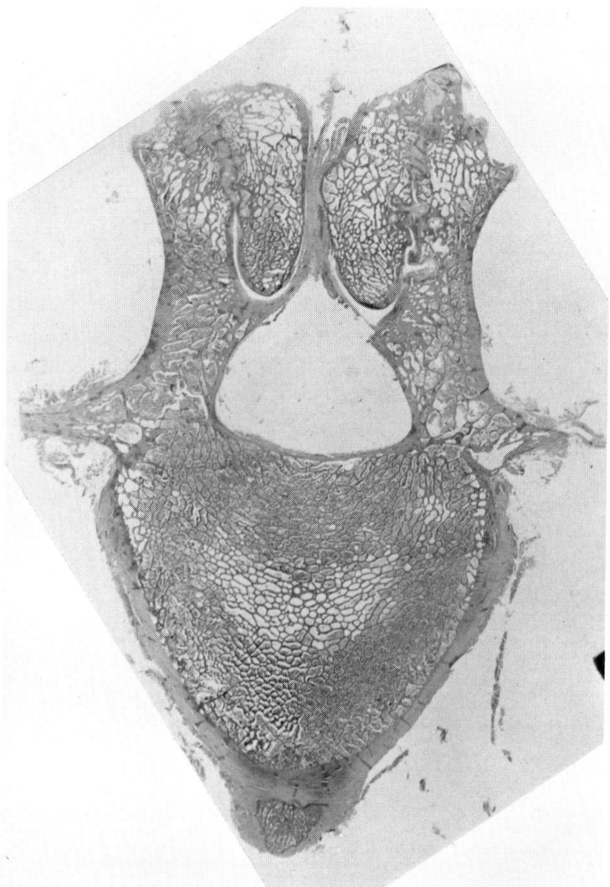

FIG. 53. Active ankylosis of the intervertebral joints between L1 and L2.

bullet will usually be found in the soft tissues ventral to the atlas. Beware of bone splinters!

Moldy corn poisoning still occurs among farm and "backyard" horses but is rare on well managed farms. The gross yellowish malacia and hemorrhages in the cerebral cortex and brain stem are readily detectable on gross examination (Fig. 52). Similar but smaller, discrete, malacic areas in the cerebral cortex have been seen as a result of septic emboli from wounds and compound fractures of the limbs.

Radiographic surveys are very useful as the preliminary step in examination of the spinal column. A variety of anatomic variations may be visualized, however, which although interesting do not relate to the clinical disease at hand.

Although "broken necks" are frequently diagnosed, they rarely occur. In the young animal (less than four or five years) there may be epiphyseal separation, usually of C2, with or without severe trauma to the spinal cord. Usually, severe overflexion of the neck results in dehiscence of the intervertebral disk and intervertebral joint ligaments with luxation and hemorrhage. Several cases of overextension (presumed) with fracture of the intervertebral articular processes have been seen. The osteochondrosis dissecans of "wobbler" may be mistaken for fractures (84).

There are three forms of spinal fusion

which usually involve the lumbar spine and occasionally the thoracic spine, but never the cervical spine: (1) The lateral transverse joints may fuse, with apparently no clinical signs. (2) The intervertebral joints may fuse. I have seen a number of such complete bony fusions at autopsy without a history of clinical signs. In one case, however, the animal, a hunter, showed pain after work over the thoracolumbar junction and distinctly resented digital pressure over this area. At autopsy L1 and L2 were actively fusing (Fig. 53). (3) There may be ventral and/or lateral bony bridging (spondylosis deformans) of two or more bodies of the lumbar and thoracic vertebrae, particularly in older horses. This may accompany severe degeneration of the intervertebral disk (uncommon) or not clearly be related to any other spinal lesions. I have not seen an example of the active stages of this process, and therefore do not know whether there are clinical signs. There are no clinical signs with the fully developed lesion.

In older horses, degeneration of the intervertebral disks is common, particularly of the cervical disks and the lumbosacral disk. Although disk degeneration is common, I have never seen disk protrusion of the type seen in, for example, man and the dog. The disk of the horse does not have a distinctly demarcated nucleus pulposus. Collagen fibers predominate throughout the disk, decreasing in concentration toward the center of the disk but still predominating over the mucoid material.

Degeneration of the equine disk consists of a gradual drying out, yellowing, and eventual disappearance of the central area.

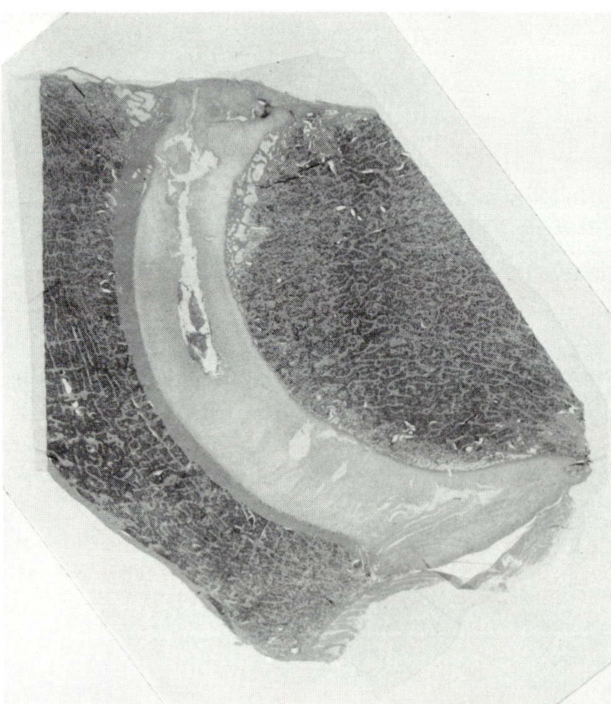

FIG. 54. Degeneration, cleft formation of a cervical intervertebral disk (toward top of photo; spaces at bottom are section artefacts).

A cleft or space remains (Fig. 54). The precise histological course of events has not been studied.

Neuritis of the cauda equina, segmental myelitis, and wobbler have been discussed elsewhere (84). A few cases of melanoma metastasizing to the vertebrae and/or spinal canal have been seen. Salmonellosis in foals may be accompanied by metastasis to and abscessation in one or more vertebrae. Large *C. equi* abscesses in the lungs may adhere to and invade the thoracic vertebrae.

The appearance of the epidural fat may be deceptive. In cachectic animals it undergoes serous atrophy, as do the other adipose tissues of the body, and the yellow-brown, gelatinous appearance may erroneously suggest an inflammatory lesion. Such changes together with multiple petechiae in the connective tissues are particularly noticeable around the cauda equina and have no local pathological significance.

Vertebral fractures and malpositions such as lordosis, scoliosis, and kyphosis have been described elsewhere (75, 84).

SIX

The Urogenital Apparatus

The order of examination of the viscera is not important. A general rule, however, is to leave the most striking lesions until last and to open the gastrointestinal tract last to avoid examining the organs in a sea of ingesta.

Dissection

Orient the urogenital block, dorsal side up, on the table. Beginning at the cranial end, open the aorta, celiac artery and its branches, the renal arteries, and the origins of the internal and external iliac arteries.

The adrenal glands are readily located in the angle formed by the medial border of the kidney, renal artery, and aorta. Examine the surface and make multiple transverse slices through the glands.

Slice the kidney from the convex border to the pelvis. The capsule can be stripped easily only if the kidney is rotten—when there is no point in doing it anyway. Nephritis will be quite apparent on the cut surface without the necessity of tearing up the cortex by stripping the capsule.

Open the ureters from the pelvis of the kidney to the urinary bladder. If difficulty is encountered in picking up the renal origin of the ureter, pick up the ureter in the angle formed by the kidney and renal artery (opposite to location of adrenal gland).

Reorient the urogenital block with the ventral surface uppermost. Open the urinary bladder along the ventral midline to the internal orifice of the urethra.

Open the intrapelvic and penile urethra of the male. The mucosa is normally intensely hyperemic in appearance. Examine and slice the seminal vesicles, prostate, and bulbourethral glands. Make multiple slices through the preputial fat, examining the superficial inguinal lymph nodes. Examine the testes, epididymes, ductus, spermatic vessels, etc. Slice the testes along the long axes and examine the cut surface.

Open the urethra of the female from the bladder into the vagina, continuing the incision along the ventral midline to open the vagina, vestibule, and vulva.

Examine the external os of the cervix for adhesions, scarring, inflammation and the like.

Open the cervix, continuing the incision through the body and both horns of the uterus. Palpate the oviducts. Examine the ovaries and slice them along the long axes into the ovulation fossae.

Open the rectum and anus along the dorsal surface. Search carefully for rectovaginal fistula (38). Slice and examine the udder and the superficial inguinal lymph nodes.

Interpretation

Urinary

Carefully examine the aorta, renal arteries and celiac artery. Numerous fibrin "tracks" may be present on the intimal surfaces (Fig. 55). These tracks are accumulations of fibrin and inflammatory cells and are easily removed by scraping the intima with a knife. They are believed (73) to represent reaction to migrating *Strongylus vulgaris* larvae.

Saddle emboli are occasionally present at the bifurcation of the aorta. Such emboli are of two distinct origins, in my experience. The first and more common is a thrombus or embolus from severe bloodworm infestation. It is noteworthy that the immature larvae in such thrombi may readily escape naked-eye detection.

The second type of embolus arises from vegetative endocarditis of the aortic valve. An animal with clinical signs of cardiac failure may suddenly become severely ataxic in the rear quarters and/or unable to stand unassisted. This results from embolization from the aortic vegetation with the embolus lodging at the aortic bifurcation.

The renal arteries are occasionally partially blocked by parasitic thrombi or emboli in cases of severe bloodworm infestation. Such blockage is usually associated with single or multiple fresh or chronic renal infarcts. If the arteries have not been examined, such infarcts may remain unexplained at the time of autopsy, and even subsequently on microscopic examination. Blockage or in-

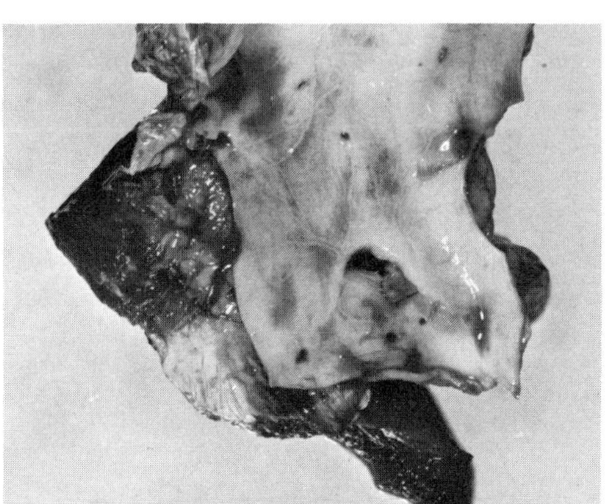

FIG. 55. Fibrin tracks on the intima of the aorta in the vicinity of the celiac artery.

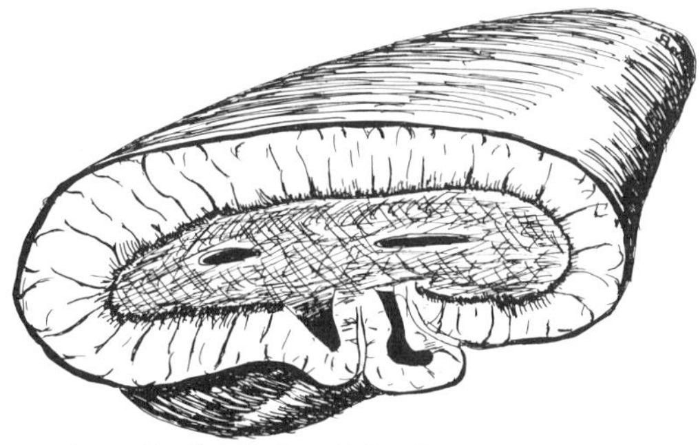

FIG. 56. Cortical nodules incorporating into the adrenal cortex.

farction of the adrenal arteries and glands has not been seen.

Medial calcification of the abdominal aorta is rare in horses as compared to cattle (54). Occasionally, one may find calcification and even ossification in and around the origin of the cranial mesenteric artery as a result of long-standing bloodworm infestation.

The adrenal cortex grows from multiple small cortical nodules (30) which are readily apparent on the capsular surface (Fig. 56). These should not be mistaken for cortical adenomas, which are rare and of considerable size. On cut section the cortex is usually a tan-gray color, shading to yellow (fatty accumulation) in animals which have been under any of a variety of "stresses." The medulla is a gray-blue color. Rarely, one may encounter a tumor mass in the medulla; this is pheochromocytoma. To my knowledge these medullary tumors are not associated with any clinical syndrome. The medullary veins are large and should not be mistaken for cystic or other pathological changes.

The inexperienced prosector frequently mistakes the normal glary, viscid, mucoid material in the renal pelvis and ureter for pus. As has been said so many times, this material is normal.

Renal lesions are uncommon but not nonexistent in horses. Occasional cases of pyelonephritis, small congenital cortical cysts (no pathological significance), and cortical abscesses (shigellosis) are seen. Glomerulonephritis has been reported (56), but I have not seen a case. In severe azoturia there may be myoglobinuric nephrosis (88). I have seen a few cases of severe hemoglobinuric nephrosis, which caused death within a week or ten days, following severe exertion in hot, humid weather. If death occurred shortly after such exertion (I have not seen an example), a red-stained, enlarged kidney would be expected. After a week, however, the kidney is enlarged and pale and the markings on the cut surface are distinctly blurred and cooked in appearance. A few cases of grossly enlarged kidneys with severe cortical hemorrhage have been seen. Histologically, there were fibrin thrombi in the glomeruli with the typical picture of acute renal cortical necrosis (Swartzman reaction). The precise pathogenesis could not, unhappily, be worked out with the histories available.

A few renal cortical adenocarcinomas have been seen in aged animals. They may cause rupture of the renal cortex with fatal bleeding. Calculi occasionally occur in older animals, may cause hydronephrosis, and are usually unilateral.

Small polypoid proliferations of the ureteral epithelium are common and not significant.

One case may be of interest because of both its rarity and the illustration of the reasonable interpretations which can be made at autopsy with relevant clinical history. Rectal examination of a stallion with severe colic revealed exquisite pain in the vicinity of the left ureter, and the veterinarian believed he palpated an enlargement in the left ureter. The pain subsided dramatically within a few hours after the rectal examination. The animal developed acute laminitis with rotation of the coffin bone and punctured soles and was destroyed five days later. At autopsy a small stone was found in the bladder and a small area of hyperemia and minimal superficial necrosis was present in the middle third of the left ureter. One may speculate that the muscular activity induced by the rectal examination had caused the stone to pass.

A greenish, sandy precipitate is quite common in the bladder, particularly in older and/or cachectic animals. Cystitis is rare, in my experience, unless there is bladder atony as the primary event. Such atony accompanies damage to the terminal portion of the spinal cord, caudal part of the lumbar enlargement, or to the sacral outflow of the parasympathetic nervous system. Segmental myelitis, sudan poisoning, and neuritis of the cauda equina are specific examples. When the carcass is first opened, the atonic bladder will appear greatly enlarged and distended with urine. Such distension may be physiological, however, and is not always pathognomonic of nerve damage.

Rupture of the urinary bladder, particularly of the dorsal surface, is not uncommon in foals, although with appropriate clinical awareness surgery is usually successful. An occasional case which is unsuspected or operated upon without discovery of a rupture does come to autopsy. Such cases are generally of two types: the rupture may be very slight, with only mild hyperemia being immediately apparent. Careful examination together with distension of the bladder will reveal pinhole tears or defects in the wall. The second type occurs as a result of invasion of the bladder wall by an abscess of the urachus, and clinical signs of septicemia and pyemia may mask the signs of leakage of urine into the peritoneal cavity.

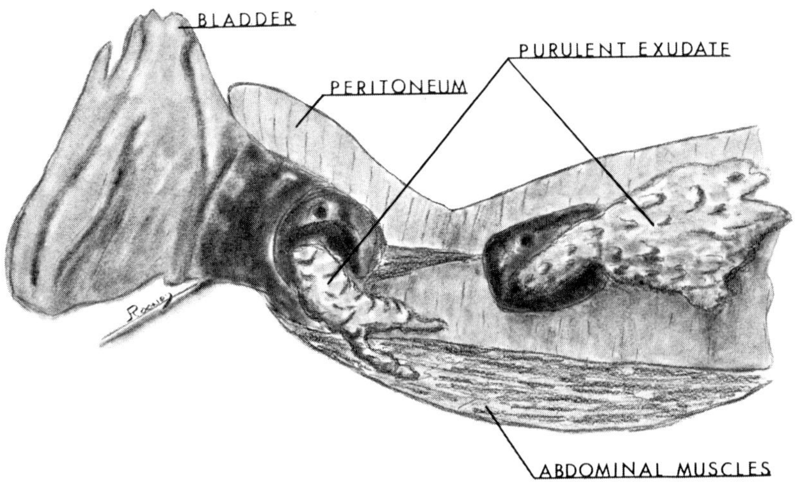

FIG. 57. Abscess of the urachus. It has been cut across and purulent material is flowing out. Urinary bladder is to the left.

Carefully examine the umbilicus and urachus of foals. The thrombotic material in the vessels is dry and yellowish and should not be mistaken for abscessation. Although dipping or painting of the umbilicus does reduce the incidence of purulent inflammation of the umbilicus, strong disinfectants such as tincture of iodine may seal the umbilicus too rapidly. Organisms which would ordinarily be flushed out by the normal weeping of the umbilical stump are sealed in and may cause an abscess of the urachus, which is not apparent on external examination and may serve as the nidus for generalized pyemia. Specifically, a foal may develop pyemia, be treated, and appear to recover only to break down repeatedly with recurrent joint infection in first one joint and then another. Such foals may have signs of a persistent urachus (dripping of urine) or appear to have a completely clean umbilicus. There are two major reasons for such recurrent cases. The first, and undoubtedly the most common, is simply that the veterinarian or owner has stopped antibiotic treatment too soon, when there is clinical evidence of recovery. The treatment must be continued for several days beyond apparent recovery in order to eliminate all organisms. If this is not done, organisms will not only persist and be able to set up a new pyemic episode but they may also be resistant to the antibiotic originally utilized.

The second case of organism persistence is the urachus abscess (Fig. 57). Often, no amount or duration of antibiotics can sterilize an abscess. It would seem justifiable to surgically explore the persistent urachus or the urachus area of a recurrent joint-ill case and remove it completely if a purulent process is apparent. This has been done in several cases with gratifying results.

Genital

Knowledge of the pathology of the reproductive tract of the male is meager (8). Testicular infection or atrophy is uncommon and obvious (the cause of the atrophy, however, is not obvious, and in my few cases has never been ascertained). In young horses small reddish plaques may be found scattered over the surface of the testis with or without adhesions to the tunica. Microscopically, these are focal accumulations of granulation tissue associated with necrotic arteries. Such arterial necrosis may be seen histologically in the absence of gross lesions, as well. The arteritis virus is not involved, and the cause is unknown. Despite the injunction to examine the accessory sex glands, I have never encountered a lesion in one of these glands. Accessory adrenal cortical tissue (small, firm, brownish masses) may be found in the tunica vaginalis of the male and near the ovary of the female.

The vestibular bulbs are frequently engorged with blood and bulge into the vagina in mares dying in shock. The vaginal mucosa is pale, white and dry-pink and moist during estrus. The remnants of the rudimentary hymen may be apparent. Complete, persistent hymen is very rare. Outbreaks of coital exanthema are occasionally seen in horse herds. The vaginal mucosa and penis are hyperemic with numerous small, yellowish pustules which burst to form erosions. The condition is self-limiting and will be seen only as an incidental lesion at autopsy.

The endometrium is grayish-red with small, soft, velvety folds. With advancing age areas of the endometrium become whiter, the folds may disappear, and there may be varying degrees of cystic change (Fig. 58): The cysts vary in size from barely visible to hen egg size. Such lesions cannot be clearly correlated with infertility.

The pregnant uterus from about 45 to 150 days has numerous, elevated, whitish-gray endometrial cups which supply nutrients to the developing embryo (Fig. 59) (104). These cups disappear as the villi form and the allantochorion implants on the endometrium (about 100 to 150 days).

Endometritis is common in mares but rarely becomes frank metritis or pyometra. There is increased reddening of the endometrium and an uneven change of the normally small amount of clear, glistening fluid to a flaky, white or yellow.

An exception is postpartum *Escherichia coli* infection. The fetus is usually aborted near term with an *E. coli* septicemia, the outstanding characteristic of which is startling hemorrhagic enteritis. All layers of the uterus will be intensely hemorrhagic with bloody fluid in the lumen. This condition can be rapidly fatal, and isolation of *E. coli* in pure culture from

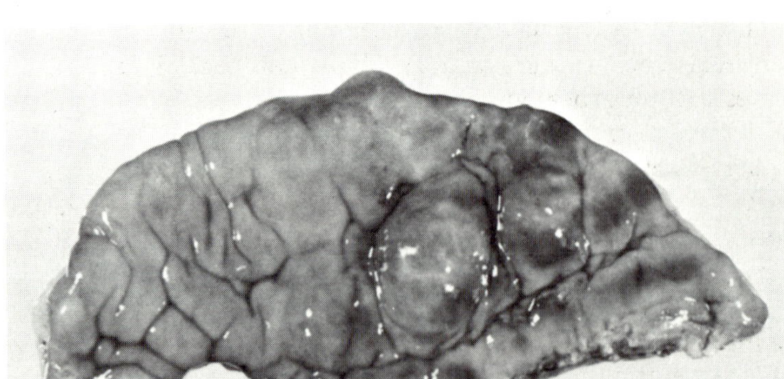

FIG. 58. Cysts in the endometrium to the right. Normal endometrium is to the left.

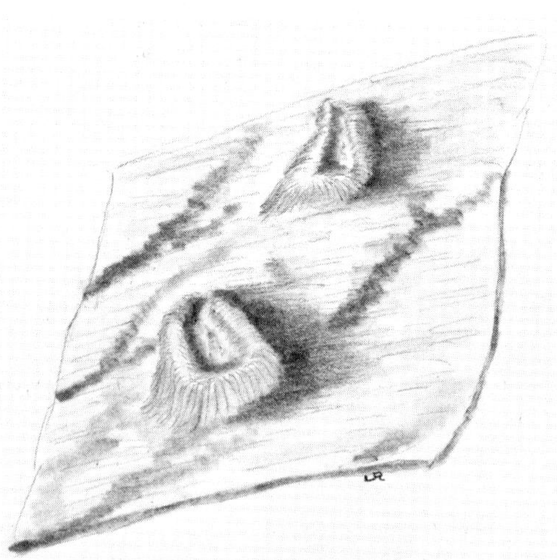

FIG. 59. Endometrial cups.

a fetus aborted near term should suggest close attention to the mare and her uterus. *E. coli* may invade the damaged reproductive organs following difficult parturition with similar results.

An occasional mare has massive pyometra with thick, yellow-white, tenacious viscid material filling and distending the uterus. The exudate may be bacteriologically and mycologically sterile—a bizarre state of affairs.

Cervicitis is a frequent clinical diagnosis. At autopsy the cervix may be hyperemic to hemorrhagic with a flaky, mucoid exudate in the presence of endometritis. I have not seen cervicitis in the absence of endometritis. Infected mares represent a major problem in equine breeding operations. There are in general two types of infected mares. The first, typically a young or maiden mare, has a normal uterus. An infectious agent, such as *Streptococcus*, *Klebsiella*, *Pseudomonas*, or *Corynebacterium* (21), is introduced by breeding, windsucking, speculum, etc. An acute endometritis develops with a marked purulent reaction. Within a few days or a week the infection is cleared by the mare's defense mechanisms, and the reproductive tract returns to a normal state (66).

The second type of mare, typically several years in the stud ranks, becomes infected during estrus. A marked inflammatory reaction does not develop. Rather, a low-grade, relatively mild reddening and sparse purulent exudate develops and persists for weeks or months. The infection may be cleared by antibiotic therapy, only to reappear during the next estrous period.

These latter mares are often dubbed "chronically infected." Evidence for this appelation is said to be the presence of a mononuclear-lymphoid cellular reaction in the endometrium. I do not feel this appelation is correct. The histological changes indicate that the uterus had been infected or had been and still is infected (if neutrophiles are present). The chronic mare does not have a chronic infection, as chronic is generally defined; rather, the defensive mechanisms are defective and an active infection is allowed to persist.

While this may appear to be nit-picking, the distinction is important. Chronic implies that the host responds to the invasion but is unable to thoroughly dispose of the invader because of the nature of the organism (fungus, acid-fast organisms, for example). Active infection, in the present context, implies that the host reaction is defective and that an organism ordinarily readily destroyed or removed is allowed to persist.

Mares with such defective defense mechanisms may become infected by almost any organism at any time. While *Streptococci* may be the most common invader, there is evidence that *Corynebacteria* are also common.

In brief, then, I feel that most serious infection problems in mares are a function of defective defense mechanisms and not a function of organism virulence. Two possible exceptions (the evidence is not completely clear as yet) are *Klebsiella* and *Pseudomonas*. Future research must provide the test for this hypothesis and perhaps an answer to the precise nature of the defective defense mechanism. Such work, happily, is in progress (66).

Localized areas of atony of the uterus have been described and considered a significant cause of infertility (52). If a fresh uterus is suspended by the cervix and tips of the horns, all degrees of atonia may be observed as rigor waxes and wanes. Thinning of the uterine wall has been described (52). When the endometrial folds disappear with age and endometrial atrophy (or simply by physically stretching the uterus at autopsy), the uterine wall will appear thinner when held up to a strong light. Both of these "states" of the uterus are either reflections of age or postmortem events and, in my experience, cannot be directly or indirectly correlated with infertility.

The only tumor encountered in the uterus has been an occasional leiomyoma in the myometrium of aged mares. This tumor can easily be overlooked unless the uterus is palpated carefully. The clinician may well be aware of this lump from rectal examination, and the prosector is indeed embarrassed if he misses it.

The oviducts have rarely, in my experience, been the site of pathological changes of any type. Only one case of unilateral hydrosalpinx has been seen (19). Parovarian cysts, remnants of the Muellerian and Wolffian ducts, are routinely found and may be of any size, from barely perceptible to fist size.

The ovaries vary considerably in size, shape, and appearance depending upon their functional state. No completely satisfactory description of the ovary can be given which will cover every ovary of every mare at every point of time. At best one can only provide general guidelines to assist the prosector in learning to evaluate properly this ever-changing and fluctuating organ.

During fetal life the gonad is quite large (it is frequently mistaken for the kidney, in fact) because of the large fetal endocrine zone. This zone occupies most of the ovary and is olive green in color. True ovarian tissue is present only as a thin, subcapsular rim. The endocrine zone gradually disappears through fetal life and at birth has almost completely disappeared. The ovary is quite small at birth but does show the future site of the ovulation fossa. Continued growth and differentiation during the first two months converts the ovary to a small adult form with a distinct ovulation fossa. The ovary increases in size gradually but is usually inactive until about one year of age. Some yearling fillies, particularly in the spring and early summer (central Kentucky), may show one or two small follicles. By two years of age the ovary has reached the full adult size and, except during midwinter, has follicular activity. From this point forward no single, general description applies to all ovaries.

At any given point in time one may find one or more follicles at various stages of development as well as corpora lutea either large and vigorous in appearance or small and apparently regressing.

In these descriptions the reader will note a tendency to describe static events as if they were being observed dynamically. I feel this is an important attribute for the prosector to develop. One can read function from structure and should always attempt to do so.

A follicle enlarges, pushing against the capsule and plunging its way through the ovary to the ovulation fossa. Depending upon the distance from the capsule at which the follicle beings to develop, there is either a marked, fluctuating bulging of the capsule or only a slight, hardly palpable, fluctuant area on the capsular surface. When the follicle ruptures into the ovulation fossa (and if it ruptures, it always does so into the fossa) (Fig. 60), the tense capsule collapses and re-expands as the cavity fills with blood. The corpora hemorrhagica bulges, button-like, into the ovulation fossa. Often strands of the fimbriated end of the oviduct will be entrapped in this button-like protrusion of the corpora hemorrhagica (see below). These strands may be differentiated from a fine network of fibrin which may lie over the button and be adherent to the walls of the fossa.

The path of the follicle from the cortex to the ovulation fossa is often tortuous and rarely completely visualized in two dimensions. The ovary must be carefully sliced in at least two planes and reconstructed in order to trace the follicular pathway (Fig. 60). In the young ovary in particular, one can by close inspection see the radial pattern of the connective tissue from the ovulation fossa to the cortex. The follicle dissects its way down these radial "roadways."

In any given ovary at any given point in time, one may see several moderate sized follicles, a corpora hemorrhagica, and one or more regressing corpora lutea.

In the pregnant mare, up to 45 or 50 days, one large corpus luteum will be

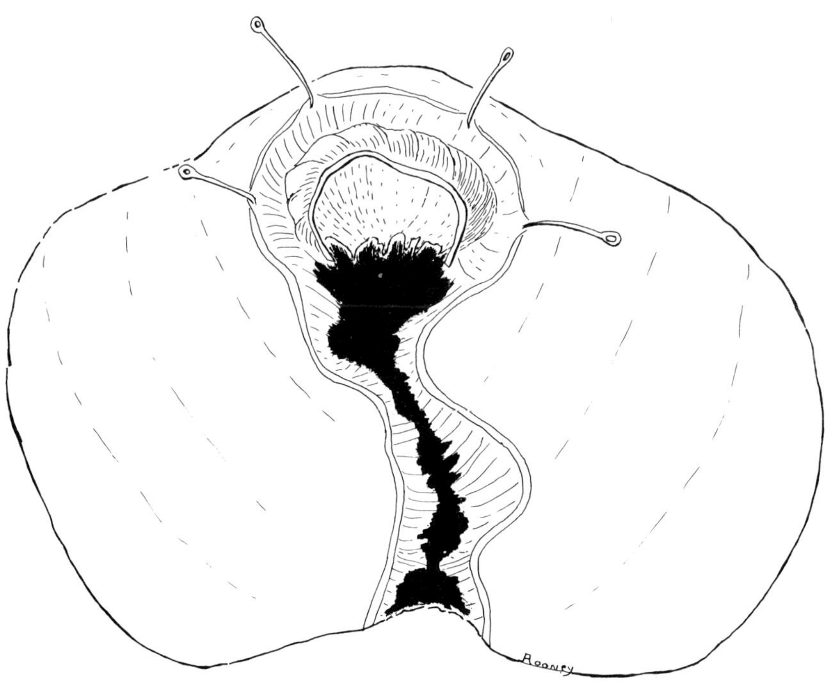

FIG. 60. Reconstruction of a recent ovulation with the track to the ovulation fossa.

present. In addition there may be regressing corpora lutea from a previous heat period as well as one or more follicles of varying size. As day 50 approaches the large corpus luteum will be regressing and numerous small follicles will be developing on one or both ovaries. After 50 days (roughly) there will be relatively few follicles and one or more corpora lutea replacing the follicles which were developing before 50 days. These corpora lutea apparently remain active until about 150 days, when they regress, and for the remainder of pregnancy one may see one or a few small follicles only.

From this description one can readily envision the many static pictures which are encountered at any given point in time. For example, assume that a mare has aborted eight to nine days before autopsy, somewhere between the 50th and 150th day of gestation. Several regressing corpora lutea will be present, and there may be one or two follicles actively developing for the "foal" heat as well as several small, inactive follicles. Ten days or so later the several small corpora lutea may be corpora albicans; there will be a large corpus luteum and perhaps a number of small follicles. With sufficient experience one can learn to read the history of recent ovarian events, but this is not easy to do and misinterpretation is frequent.

One frequently encounters small, luteinized foci close to the ovulation fossa. Their nature is unclear. They may be atretic follicles which have undergone luteinization. On the other hand, small follicles may ovulate, releasing eggs and luteinizing. Such "minor" ovulations may be the source of the numbers of eggs which can frequently be recovered from the oviducts (19, 101).

As the mare ages the pieces of fimbria entrapped and drawn into the tissue of the ovulation fossa as succeeding generations of corpora hemorrhagica contract may form inclusion cysts in greater or lesser numbers. These cysts are distinguishable grossly from follicles by their location, smaller size, and the white, opaque cyst lining. Follicles, on the other hand, generally have a glistening, finely pink, velvety lining with the perifollicular blood vessels showing through. A magnifying lens is of obvious help in such evaluations.

It is reasonable to assume that these inclusion cysts contribute to infertility in the older mare. The follicle must work its way around and through a labryinthine mass of inclusion cysts to reach the ovulation fossa. The movement of the ovum down this tortuous pathway may be so delayed that the ovum is nonviable by the time it reaches the oviduct.

The clinical diagnosis of follicular cysts or cystic ovaries is extremely difficult to validate or deny at autopsy. The clearest case is the grossly enlarged ovary (one only) which, on section, is a multiloculated cystic mass containing either golden yellow and/or bloody fluid. The cysts are lined by brownish-pink tissue and microscopically the mass is clearly a granulosa cell tumor, the only tumor that has been found in the mare's ovary.

Since any given ovary may have a variety of follicles of varying size at any given time, it is impossible at the static moment of autopsy to say, "This is a cystic ovary!" Cystic ovary in the mare is, in my opinion, a misnomer for a clinical entity (only determinable clinically) which might better be called follicular retention or detention syndrome.

The clinician may palpate an ovary serially and find a number of follicles developing simultaneously or one after the other. With regularly repeated palpation, it becomes apparent that these follicles are persisting for a considerable period of time and/or being joined by newly developing follicles until the ovary is a mass of follicles of varying sizes. These findings may be accompanied by heat abnormalities such as prolonged, aberrant heat or no heat.

If this ovary is examined in the autopsy room, one cannot say that it is cystic but only that it has a number of follicles of healthy, normal appearance. Giant follicles are very uncommon. The clinical impression of a very large follicle may be the result of the inability of the palpating fingers to distinguish, through the wall of the rectum, several normally sized follicles, and the clinician feels that he is palpating one large follicle. The tough, thick ovarian capsule obviously compounds this problem of differentiation at arm's length.

The pathologist, then, cannot confirm a diagnosis of cystic ovary but can only concur that there are numerous follicles in the ovary. Only the clinician can know whether those follicles have been there "too long." In support of this is the simple fact that eventually such ovaries return to normal, probably as the numerous follicles undergo atresia.

Having gone to such lengths on this topic it would seem apropos to suggest a cause for such follicular retention syndrome. Perhaps a sufficiently dense mass of inclusion cysts could prevent ovulation altogether and result in a "piling up" of follicles. This is completely out of my realm, but it seems possible that a deficiency of luteinizing hormone, for whatever reason, could result in many follicles reaching the ovulatory stage without the process of ovulation being initiated. Beyond these speculations I cannot proceed.

Rupture of one of the uterine or pelvic arteries is a cause of fatal or severe postpartum hemorrhage in the older mare. The iliac arteries have already been considered. The most common site is the uterine artery of the pregnant horn (Fig. 61). In very old mares the ovarian artery may rupture at about the seventh month of gestation. Copper deficiency has been suggested, on extremely tenuous grounds, as the cause of such ruptures. It seems that the advanced ages to which mares are bred is a much more likely cause. The cumulative effect of multiple pregnancies over many years and the gradually accruing effects of senility finally culminate in arterial rupture (80). It is doubtful whether any single element or factor will be the cause. As in so many other aspects of pathology, multiple factors are undoubtedly operating.

Pale white or lemon-yellow subcutaneous tissue immediately suggests internal hemorrhage. When the abdomen is opened, large quantities of nonclotted blood flow out. The site of the rupture may be indicated by the position of the partially clotted hematoma: retroperitoneal with internal or external iliac artery rupture; cranial part of the broad ligament with ovarian artery rupture; and the middle or whole broad ligament when the uterine artery is ruptured.

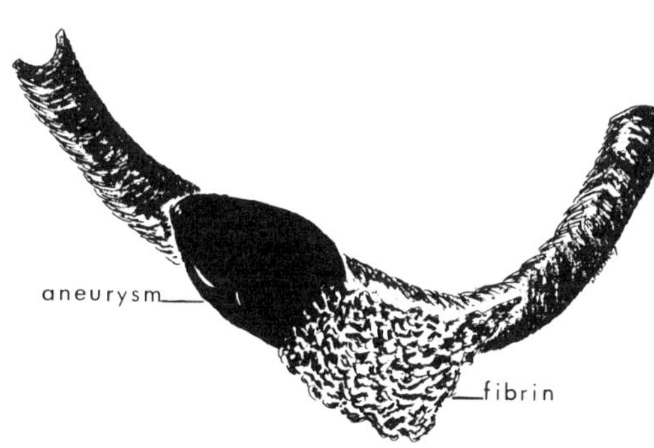

FIG. 61. Bulging (berry) aneurysm of the uterine artery. The aneurysm has ruptured and fibrin masses are present at and near the rupture site.

With care the site of the rupture of the broad ligament releasing blood into the abdominal cavity can be discerned. It appears that the initial bleeding fills and distends the broad ligament, with acute clinical signs being present at this time. For a time the broad ligament may hold and remain intact, and the clinical signs of hemorrhagic shock abate. If the bleeding continues, the broad ligament eventually ruptures, spilling blood into the peritoneal cavity with an immediate reappearance of acute and terminal signs of hemorrhagic shock.

For the novice the best procedure for locating the site of the vessel rupture is to orient the urogenital block dorsal side up, locate the origins of the ovarian and uterine arteries, and carefully follow them distad until the rupture site is located. With experience one may bluntly dissect into the largest point of the hematoma and quickly locate variable-sized masses of dry, granular, brownish fibrin. These masses are always close to and/or adherent to the rupture site, and by carefully dissecting around them with the fingers the vessel and rupture site can be quickly located.

Occasionally, one may either clinically or at autopsy encounter a brownish, dry, encapsulated mass in one broad ligament. This is an organizing hematoma dating from a previous parturition and should not be mistaken for a tumor, abscess, or aberrant strongyle lesion.

SEVEN

The Spleen, Liver, Pancreas, and Duodenum

Dissection

Examine the spleen, splenic lymph nodes, vessels, and associated nerves. Make multiple transverse slices and examine the cut surfaces.

With the visceral surface of the liver up, open the descending duodenum and examine the orifices of the common bile duct and pancreatic duct (diverticulum duodeni) and the accessory pancreatic duct. Slice and examine the pancreas.

Separate the pancreas and duodenum from the liver. Examine the hepatic lymph nodes. Open the major radicles of the portal vein and bile duct.

Turn the liver over, examine the diaphragmatic surface, examine the lining of the caudal vena cava, open the major branches of the hepatic veins, and slice the liver thoroughly.

Interpretation

Spleen

Indentations of the capsule of the lateral surface of the head of the spleen are common and normal. They will be more obvious and striking if the spleen is distended with blood (acute splenic swelling). Pinpoint reddish protrusions of splenic pulp through defects in the capsule are also common and normal. Pentobarbital euthanasia, acute septicemia, and lightning stroke may be accompanied by acute splenic swelling. Splenic enlargement, in fact, is a lesion of primary shock, whether caused by septicemia, electrical shock, anesthesia, or something else. The spleen will tend to be smaller than average and apparently fibrotic in older animals (senile splenic atrophy). Accessory splenic tissue may be present in the greater omentum and/or the gastrosplenic ligament.

The spleen is for me a singularly unenlightening organ. One can learn very little from this organ, either grossly or microscopically.

Pancreas and Duodenum

In the foal intense hyperemia of the duodenal mucosa is suggestive of *Strongyloides* sp. infestation. Such infestations are apparently of little or no clinical significance. *Gasterophilus nasalis* may be present in the first part of the duodenum. The rare case of hemorrhagic pancreatitis may be caused by migration of strongyle larvae (*S. equinus*, *S. edentatus*). There will be fresh bleeding, edema, and frank discoloration of the pancreatic parenchyma. Interstitial edema, accumulation of blood, and blackish (H_2S) discoloration of the pancreas are common postmortem decomposition lesions and must not be confused with true pancreatitis.

I have seen two cases of severe, massive destruction and fibrosis of the pancreas and liver. Although no larvae were found, the microscopic sections strongly suggested parasitic migration, presumably of *S. equinus*. A similar case has been reported (5).

Pure, yellowish edema fluid around the pancreas and in the sublumbar retroperitoneal tissues suggests lesions in the chest (heart, pleuritis). We shall digress at this point to consider equine viral arteritis. The gross autopsy findings have been described (49):

"Edema, congestion, and hemorrhage, the most prominent gross manifestations, were related both in intensity and frequency to lesions in arteries of microscopic size. . . . The subcutaneous tissues at the sites of inoculation were generally edematous and congested, the edema extending ventrally along the fascia. Edema of the subcutis was often prominent in the legs below the knees or hocks.

"In the digestive system, the oral cavity and esophagus were unaffected, but congestion and petechiae were seen in the pharynx and glandular part of the stomach. The small intestine was severely involved by edema and congestion of the mucosa and submucosa, usually most intense in segments of intestine 1 to 6 feet in length, which alternated with sections of relatively normal appearance. The crests of the mucosal folds were especially congested and glistened with an excessive amount of mucus. In the crowded intestine submucosal edema was most conspicuous in the submucosa of the ventral colon and apex of the cecum. In most cases submucosal edema also extended from the origin of the anterior mesenteric artery along the course of the cecal and colic arteries. In some animals which had exhibited diarrhea, the mucosa of the large intestine was blood red except where it was covered by adherent feces-stained membranes. Removal of these membranes disclosed a raw surface beneath.

"In the respiratory system the mucous membrane of the pharynx, larynx, trachea, and guttural pouches were congested and contained many petechiae. The weight of the lungs was increased because of the edema which thickened the subpleural and interlobular septa, particularly along the ventral margins and in the apex. Emphysema was frequent, especially at the apex and along the margins of the cardiac notch, giving the pleural surface an uneven, 'knobby' appearance. Congestion and petechiae were common, and the subpleural lymphatics were often dilated. The major bronchi usually contained more than the normal amount of mucus.

"The gross changes in the heart were variable. In some cases only a few petechiae and some edema were noted in the fat at the base of the heart; in others, subendocardial hemorrhages were particularly prominent around the valves. Generally the myocardium appeared paler than normal, and in one case the right heart was dilated. The pericardium was often congested and the adjacent mediastinum edematous.

"The spleen in most cases was neither enlarged nor turgid, but in a few mares it was greatly enlarged and turgid from engorgement with dark, partially congealed blood. Hemorrhagic infarcts were observed in spleens from both fetuses and adult horses.

"In the kidneys the cortex was pale in contrast to the dark, congested medulla. The perirenal tissues were infiltrated by edema in nearly all cases.

"The lymph nodes that were edematous but not conspicuously enlarged were seen most consistently in the mediastinum and mesentery. The mesenteric lymph nodes in animals with enteritis exhibited severe congestion and hemorrhages.

"In pregnant mares experimentally infected, the wall of the uterus was thickened with edema, which was particularly prominent in the subserosa and near the attachment of the broad ligament. In some cases the uterus contained a dead fetus; in others, abortion had occurred before the mare died.

"The changes about the eyes consisted of congestion and edema of the conjunctiva with occasional petechiae. The cornea had assumed a milky opalescence, and in a few cases the aqueous humor was cloudy."

It should be emphasized that the lesions described were seen in experimental cases. The few natural outbreaks observed in the United States have caused clinical signs (fever, stocking-up, brickred mucosae) as well as abortion in pregnant mares, but no deaths in postnatal animals have been reported.

Liver

Lesions are uncommon in the portal vein. Rarely, a fibrin track may be seen (aberrant *S. vulgaris*?). Pigment stones are occasionally seen in the bile duct and have little significance except to indicate cachexia.

Variability in the size of the liver lobes is common. In particular, atrophy of the right lobe of the liver occurs in older horses. The atrophy begins at the free, ventral border and progresses dorsally to eventually involve the caudate lobe. The usual explanation (16) for this atrophy, continuous pressure by the large intestine, is not satisfying, but there is no better explanation to offer at this time.

Variable numbers of fibrous tags, white or pinkish-white in color, are invariably present on the diaphragmatic surface of the left lobe of the liver in every adult horse (Fig. 62) (perihepatitis filamentosa). Occasionally they stretch as bands from the capsule of the liver to the diaphragm and may be associated with variable-sized plaques of capsular fibrosis. There may be a few such tags on the middle and right lobes. These lesions are not associated with changes in the underlying liver parenchyma, and the cause is not known. Since *S. edentatus* larvae preferentially migrate through the right lobe of the liver, it is, perhaps unreasonable to ascribe the tags and scars to such migrations. There is no evidence that this localized peritonitis is associated with a clinical syndrome, either in the acute or chronic stages.

It is manifestly impossible to present a complete course in liver pathology in the space available, and we must restrict ourselves to some common, obvious points. Telangiectasia and the small focal fatty infarcts so commonly seen in cattle are extremely rare in horses. The extrahepatic biliary system may be virtually eliminated from consideration. I do not mean that this system should not be examined; the rarity of lesions makes it mandatory that it be carefully examined. Considering

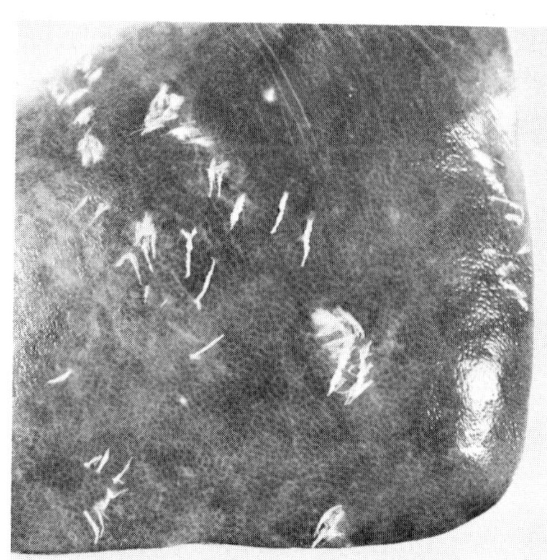

FIG. 62. Fibrous tags (perihepatitis filamentosa) on the diaphragmatic surface of the liver.

the liver itself, the first and most important determination is the extent of postmortem decomposition. There is no way to describe this accurately. Only experience will clearly reveal to the prosector the difference between a true lesion and focal or diffuse rot. In general, a diffuse, clay-tan color, soft, floppy consistency, and blurred, murky appearance of the cut surface characterize rot. In a fresh carcass this appearance is justifiably dubbed cloudly swelling and indicates that the animal was running a high fever and/or subjected to a severe septicemic or toxic process. One must be very careful in making such a distinction, however, because the early stages of rot are identical with those of cloudy swelling.

An animal dying of right side heart failure or pleuritis will have passive congestion of the liver. The centers of the lobules will be dark and blood-filled whereas the periphery will be pale or tan. Similarly, in shock, severe toxemia, or septicemia the circulatory system fails, and there will be an irregularly distributed passive congestion of the liver.

Gross fatty degeneration of the liver is not common in horses but is frequently seen in ponies. It is indicated most clearly by rounding of the normally sharp liver borders. A distinct yellow color is rarely seen except in exceptionally obese ponies.

Small, discrete fibrous and/or calcified nodules are encountered with some frequency either deep in the parenchyma or bulging on the capsular surface. These are the scarred remnants of parasitic migrations.

Focal or diffuse fibrosis (cirrhosis) of the liver has not been common in my experience. *Senecio* or other plant poisonings lead to diffuse fibrosis (liver-brain syndrome). I have seen two cases of severe liver fibrosis and atrophy as a result of complete or nearly complete thrombosis of the hepatic artery caused by *S. vulgaris* larvae. Focal areas of apparent fibrosis in an atrophic right liver lobe are, in fact, collapsed and condensed connective tissue framework brought about by atrophy of the parenchyma.

Careful study of the lobular architecture on the cut surface may reveal the presence of amyloid—a homogenized, smooth appearance within the lobules. With the exception of serum-production horses amyloidosis is not nearly so common in the horse as textbook descriptions might suggest.

The cellular infiltrates of equine infectious anemia localize, particularly, adjacent to the portal areas as white bands or discrete masses. Equine infectious anemia has been well described pathologically (16, 28, 100). The animal which dies naturally will usually show severe anemia and icterus whereas the animal which is destroyed will not. The liver may not be enlarged but will be heavier and stiffer than normal.

In Theiler's disease, or serum hepatitis (98), there is massive, acute necrosis of virtually every liver cell. Grossly, the liver lobules, both on the capsular and cut surface, are yellowish or whitish with, in some cases, a distinct, greenish cast.

Acute hepatic toxins of any type may produce grossly apparent zones of gray-white necrosis within the hepatic lobules. Such a distinction is difficult to make, however, because both the passive congestion of specific or nonspecific circulatory failure and postmortem decomposition (cloudy swelling) can cause the same appearance. Microscopic examination is necessary.

EIGHT

The Gastrointestinal Tract

Dissection

Spread out the great mesentery and the mesocolon and examine them. Slice the mesenteric lymph nodes.

Carefully open the stomach along the greater curvature, laying the flap over and noting the layering of the ingesta in the stomach. Remove the ingesta and note the odor, color, and consistency. Examine the mucosa.

Open the small intestine with knife or scissors along the antimesenteric attachment.

Lay out the large intestine with the medial surface upward. Sever the cecocolic ligament. Examine the chains of colic and cecal lymph nodes. Open the cranial mesenteric artery and all its branches, noting the autonomic nerves and the veins accompanying the arteries (Fig. 63).

Open the ileum into the cecum, examining the ileocecal valve (93). Open the cecum from the base to apex. Locate the cecocolic orifice and open the ventral, dorsal, and descending colons.

Interpretation

Movements of the Intestine

Postmortem and agonal changes are rife and overlapping, and cause untold difficulties for the novice prosector. One may learn a great deal about the interpretation of the gastrointestinal tract by watching the changes which occur in a freshly killed animal (2).

The stomach does not move and movement cannot be elicited by mechanical stimulation. The small intestine is always moving and may continue to move for at least one-half hour. Segmenting and pendular movements are readily seen and short peristaltic rushes may be observed. Mechanical stimulation (knife point) easily induces movement. The large intestine is usually moving or can be stimulated to move. The cecum and ventral and dorsal colon show segmenting movements which may propagate for a short distance. The descending colon does not move and stimulation is rarely effective. The large intestine movements usually disappear before the small intestine movements (roughly 15 minutes). If one assumes that death immediately disrupts the coordinating activities of the extrinsic autonomic innervation, it is apparent that the stomach and descending colon are dependent upon the extrinsic nerves. The cecum and dorsal and ventral colon are somewhat less dependent, and the small intestine is least dependent upon extrinsic nerves. Since no long peristaltic rushes are ever observed in the small intestine after death, however, such rushes may be dependent upon extrinsic nerve coordination of the intrinsic motility of the small intestine.

Eventually all motility is lost as the

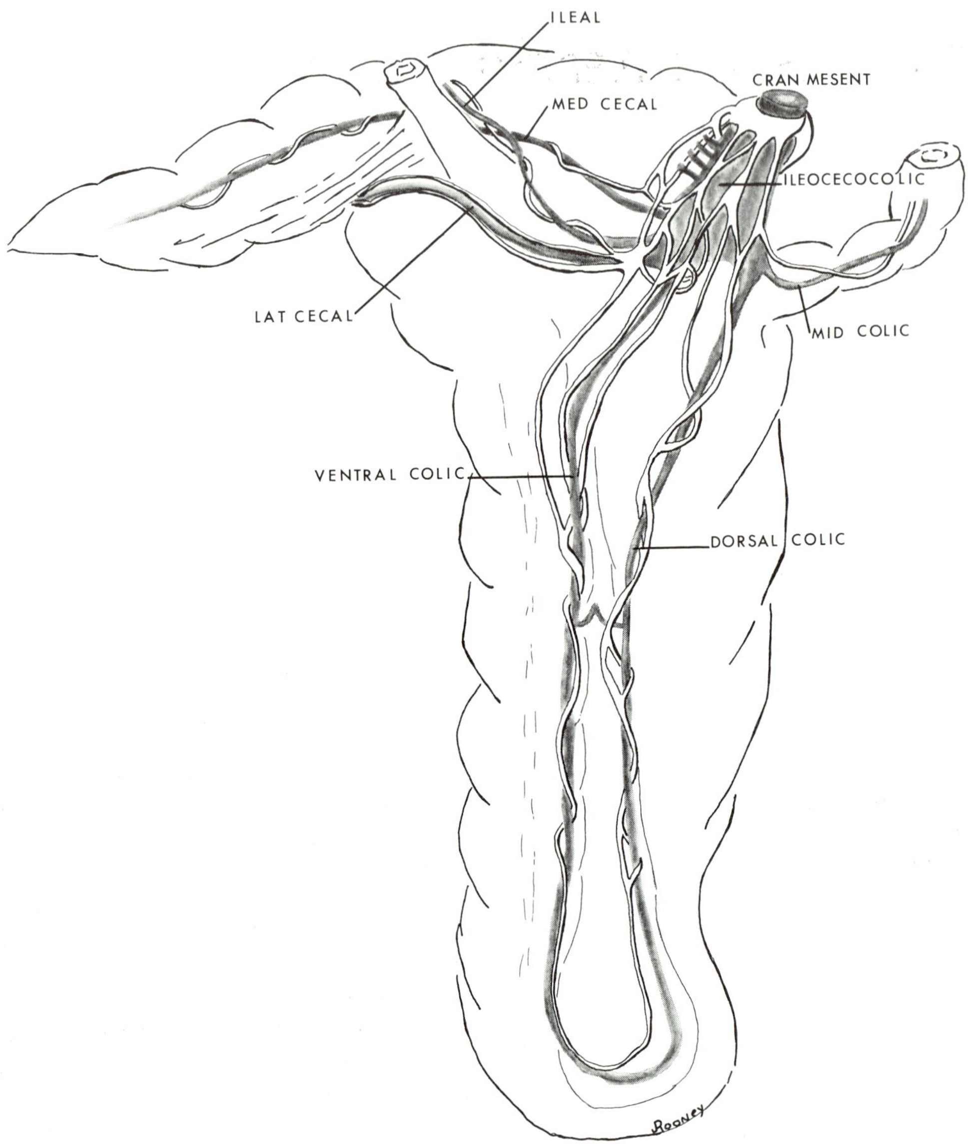

FIG. 63. Arteries and nerves of the large intestine. Only the medial portion of the course of the lateral cecal artery is shown.

intestine goes into rigor. Rigor is usually quite obvious in the small intestine but much less so in the large intestine. Rigor disappears in a short time, and the intestinal wall becomes flabby. During the agonal period the intestine moved. After death (other than destroying the animal) there is probably very little, if any, movement. Rigor comes and goes. Decomposition sets in quickly. One can easily see that a variety of vascular changes and color patterns can be produced.

The circulatory system fails during the agonal period and blood will be shunted about passively by intestinal movements. Similarly, rigor will squeeze blood about passively, particularly into the mucosal folds and tips of villi. As rigor wanes, the more dependent loops of intestine in particular (the down side) will fill with fluid and mucus while blood passively leaks out of vessels and works into the tissues, hemolyzing and diffusing. This postmortem hypostatic staining will be most obvious (and occur first) in dependent, distended loops of bowel.

Pure antemortem hyperemia (passive, agonal shunting) will appear as a diffuse bright-red color. Pure postmortem "hypermia" appears as distinct arborization of blood vessels with a diffuse, reddish staining of the immediately adjacent tissues. "Real" inflammatory antemortem hypermia appears as multiple, fine petechiae. From a distance the petechiae may have the fused appearance of pure antemortem hyperemia. Close inspection will show the petechiae.

It is known that water and food materials pass very rapidly from the stomach to the cecum. Water will appear at a cecal fistula within 15 to 20 minutes after ingestion. The following observations may be used to construct a hypothesis for a part of the mechanics of the equine digestive tract. I emphasize that this is a hypothesis.

When the small intestine is opened, it will either be empty or, if it contains food material, hay or grass will be present primarily as isolated boluses scattered at random throughout the length of the small intestine. If the animal died immediately after a large feeding of grass, there may be quantities throughout the intestine and the bolus formation may be somewhat less apparent.

If the animal has recently eaten a quantity of grain, the grain will be loosely scattered throughout the small intestine, rarely appearing as boluses.

As is well known, food materials accumulate in discrete layers in the stomach.

The hypothesis is that because food material accumulates in layers in the stomach, a differential rate of passage through the small intestine is permitted. When roughage reaches the pylorus, a signal (unspecified) is produced which causes the roughage to move rapidly to the cecum (30 minutes). During this rapid passage the readily soluble nutrients are absorbed. Since cellulose digestion must proceed in the cecum and ventral colon, however, the bulk is moved rapidly through the small intestine in order to arrive where it will be digested. When a layer of grain reaches the pylorus, a different signal (or perhaps no signal) is produced, so that the grain passes slowly along the small intestine, allowing fat, protein, and soluble sugars to be digested and absorbed.

The cecum and ventral colon absorb primarily cellulose digestion products, largely short-chain fatty acids, whereas the dorsal colon and descending colon appear to be concerned mainly with water reabsorption.

One may use this hypothesis to suggest some part of the pathogenesis of laminitis after excessive ingestion of water and/or grain. During exercise the intestinal tract is quiet. If water is given immediately after exercise, the stomach could be quickly flushed out, with mixed grain and roughage traveling rapidly to the cecum. A sudden flood of cold water into the stomach could cause a muscular spasm of the stomach in addition to the simple flushing mechanism. The sudden appearance in the cecum of large quantities of soluble carbohydrate and protein, which should have been digested and absorbed in the small intestine could encourage bacterial action on the proteins (bacterial flora shift?), resulting in the production of a variety of toxic amines.

Simple overeating of grain can lead to laminitis, and once again one may envision a simple overloading or saturation of the differential mechanism, so that grain arrives in the cecum before sufficient digestion has taken place in the small intestine.

Large Intestine

As the large intestine is opened note the character of the ingesta before removal. The ingesta are quite watery in the cecum, are progressively drier through the ventral and dorsal colons and very dry in the descending colon. Any change in this normal gradient is indicative of pathological change. Dry cecal content indicates ileus of this part only and is often accompanied by thickening of the cecal wall (see below).

Focal dry ingesta at any point may be accompanied by thickening of the wall (chronic obstipation) or a normal wall (acute obstipation) (see below, *Chronic Colic*). General dryness of the ingesta is present in shaker foal, botulism, Theiler's disease, and indeed in any severe, dehydrating process. Interestingly, it appears that in severe dehydration water is removed from the large intestine and appears in large quantities in the small intestine. However, when this situation is encountered, one must be wary and search for a lesion (intussusception, strangulation, etc.) in the area of the ileum which prevents movement of fluid and ingesta from the small to the large intestine.

General fluidity of the large intestine is seen in severe, acute diarrheas (salmonella, exhaustion shock) and in that poorly defined disease, chronic diarrhea.

After the ingesta have been removed the numerous solitary lymphoid nodules in the mucosa-submucosa will be apparent. They decrease in size and number with age. Fine petechiation of the mucosa is a common primary shock lesion.

Tapeworms, *Anoplocephala perfoliata*, may be found in moderate numbers attached to the mucosa in the vicinity of the ileocecal and cecocolic orifices (Fig. 64). At the present time, they do not appear to have any pathogenetic significance. Adult large strongyles are readily observed attached to the mucosa of the cecum and colon. Small strongyles, which may be present in large numbers, can only be seen by careful examination and magnification.

Solitary abscesses are occasionally encountered in the wall of the large intestine. With the exception of *Corynebacterium equi*, these lesions are generally of such age and contamination (as a result of ulceration into the lumen) that neither culture nor section provides any real clue as to the original cause. These abscesses may cicatrize with age, causing gradual stenosis or segmental ileus. *C. equi* ulceration and abscessation of the colon and

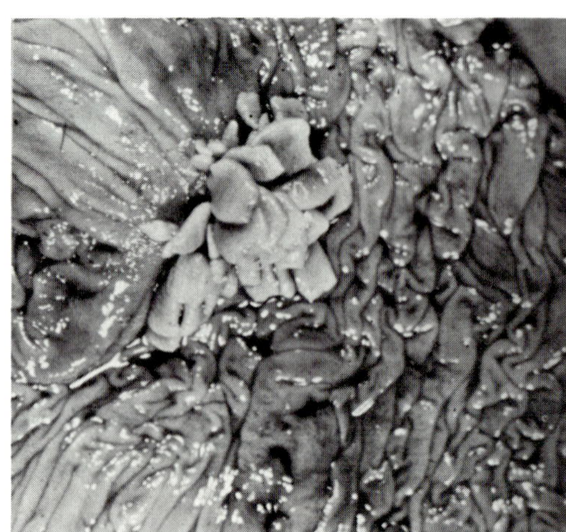

FIG. 64. *Anoplocephala perfoliata* attached to cecal mucosa close to the ileocecal orifice.

regional lymph nodes are seen in foals, although in my experience the pneumonic form has been much more common.

Salmonellosis (13, 14) is an epizootic disease of young foals on certain premises and an isolated disease of older horses under some form of "stress" (surgery, chronic disease, worming). In the acute fulminant case, death may occur within hours after onset of the disease, and the serosa of the entire large intestine shows severe hyperemia and fine petechiation. The ingesta are thin and watery and may be yellowish or blood-tinged. Evidence of diarrhea may have been noted on external examination but in peracute cases it may be absent. The mucosa is intensely congested and hemorrhagic, particularly in the cecum and ventral colon. Fulminant cases are not readily differentiated from exhaustion shock. In somewhat less fulminant cases variable ulcerations in the solitary lymphoid nodules will be seen on careful and close examination. In more prolonged cases frank abscessation of the lymphoid nodules will be apparent, and the mucosal hyperemia will be somewhat less intense and localized around the abscessed nodules. Both cultures and sections are indicated. The histological picture may be quite characteristic even though cultures are negative.

Exhaustion shock is a sporadic, peracute, and highly fatal disease of the horse (77). It is characterized by the sudden onset of severe diarrhea and toxemia or by the sudden onset of severe gastrointestinal distension (flatulence, gas colic). The temperature may be normal or elevated during the early phase, becoming normal or subnormal as the condition progresses. Limited blood studies indicate there are hemoconcentration and leukopenia (white blood cell count of less than 4,000). Dehydration occurs rapidly in both the diarrheal and nondiarrheal forms.

Toxemia appears with the onset of symptoms: depression; muddy, discolored mucous membranes; weak, thready, rapid pulse; patchy sweating; dyspnea; and cramping abdominal pains. The animal dies within 3 to 24 hours after onset despite intravenous fluid and steroid therapy. Heavy, continued steroid therapy appears to delay the fatal termination and may have allowed recovery in a few animals.

Horses of all ages appear to be susceptible, although most of my cases have been in the 1- to 10-year-old range. Cases have been seen in animals over 20 years, but only one equivocal case has been diagnosed in a suckling foal. The condition is definitely sporadic and noncontagious. Single cases may appear at any time of the year and under all types of environmental and management conditions.

The carcass is dehydrated and the subcutaneous blood vessels are engorged with dark, tarry, nonclotting blood. Petechiae and ecchymoses appear in the subcutaneous tissues of the neck and chest.

The cecum and colon have a dull, reddish-blue, cyanotic appearance on the serosal surface. There is a large quantity of fluid, often foamy, and odoriferous ingesta. The distended cecum-colon and fluid content are readily apparent as the viscera are removed from the abdominal cavity.

The mucosal lesions vary in intensity from hyperemia with fine petechiae apparent in a dull, plum-red background to a greenish-black, intensely hemorrhagic necrosis. The submucosa is often severely edematous and, less frequently, hemorrhagic (Fig. 65). There is rarely free blood in the contents.

In general, the lesions are most severe in the cecum and ventral colon, fading to the normal gray-white color at some point

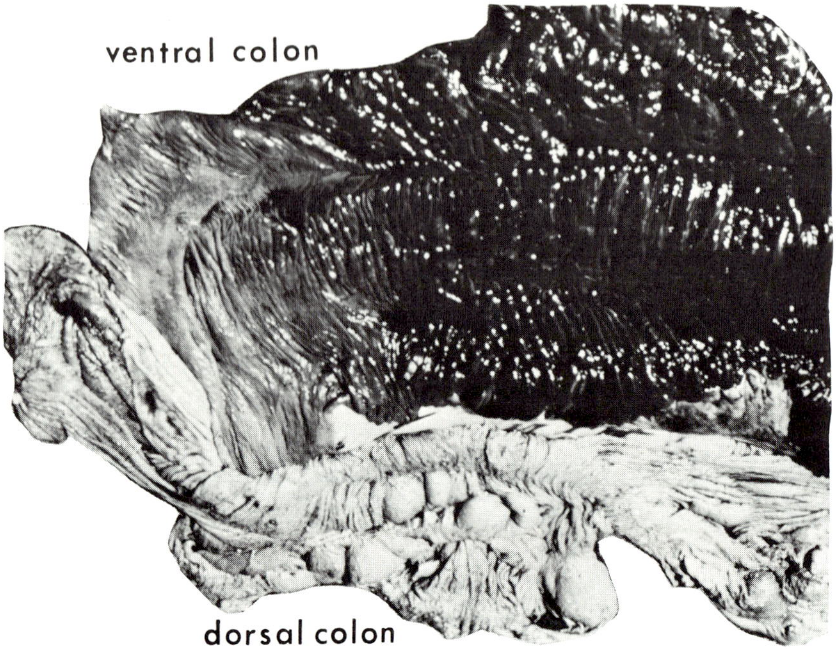

FIG. 65. Exhaustion shock. The ventral colon is intensely edematous and engorged with blood while the dorsal colon is normal.

between the pelvic flexure and transverse colon. Variations are: involvement of the cecum only, ventral colon only, and dorsal and ventral colon only. Variable degrees of hyperemia are apparent in the ileum and first part of the descending colon. The cecocolic lymph nodes are hyperemic and edematous.

No significant lesions are found in the stomach, duodenum, jejunum, pancreas, or urogenital tract. The liver is on occasion somewhat enlarged and bluish with dark, nonclotting blood running out on section. The spleen is normal or slightly enlarged with a dark-red or black color and loss of follicular markings on section. The adrenal glands routinely have patchy or massive cortical hemorrhages.

The lungs have alveolar emphysema and hyperemia and, on occasion, moderate edema. Petechiation of the parietal pleura of the thoracic wall and diaphragm is common; ecchymosis is somewhat less common.

The heart appears normal or flabby, and symmetrically or asymmetrically (right side) dilated with a grayish, "cooked" appearance on section. Epicardial petechiae and ecchymosis of the left ventricular myocardium are usually present.

Varying degrees of hyperemia, petechiation, and ecchymosis are found in the trachea, nasal passages, guttural pouches, and sinuses.

Selye's (92) concept of the general adaptation syndrome will be used as the basis for discussion of the cause of this condition. The general adaptation syndrome consists of three phases: the alarm reaction, which is subdivided into shock and countershock; the stage of resistance; and the stage of exhaustion.

The shock phase is considered comparable to so-called "primary shock." Numerous examples of death in primary shock, or the shock phase of the alarm reaction, are available in equine pathology. Electrical shock or lightning strike causes death instantly or within minutes. Spinal shock, resulting from fractures and massive hemorrhage into the spinal canal, may cause death very rapidly. In neither of these cases are lesions (other than fine mucosal petechiae) of the large intestine observed. Anesthetic shock, another example of primary shock, similarly does not result in significant lesions of the large intestine.

Hemorrhagic shock in parturient mares is particularly instructive. Some mares show clinical evidence of shock shortly after foaling and die within a matter of hours. Other mares appear to recover after the initial shock period (countershock) only to lapse again within hours and die. In neither case do lesions of the large intestine appear.

Anaphylactic shock in the horse has not been adequately described. On the basis of two fatal experimental cases, it appears that the lesions are similar in type but different in distribution from those of exhaustion shock. There is severe edema and hemorrhage throughout the gastrointestinal tract. There is severe alveolar emphysema associated with bronchiolar spasm and distinct right-side cardiac dilatation. The precise relationship of anaphylactic and exhaustion shock must await further studies.

Selye (92) has stated:

"The stage of resistance represents the sum of all non-specific systemic reactions elicited by prolonged exposure to stimuli to which the organism has acquired adaptation. It is mainly characterized by an increased resistance to the particular stressor agent to which the body has been exposed and a decrease resistance to other stimuli.

"The stage of exhaustion represents the sum of all non-specific systemic reactions which ultimately develop as a result of prolonged over-exposure to stimuli to which adaptation has been developed but could no longer be maintained."

The hypothesis is that colitis *X*, or exhaustion shock, is in reality comparable to the exhaustion phase of the general adaptation syndrome.

Evidence will now be adduced to support this hypothesis. It was recognized that many, although not all, of the animals dying with lesions of exhaustion shock had a history of a "stressing" situation 10 days to 2 weeks earlier. The concept of a silent period between the original stress and the onset of exhaustion shock developed. The concept was vulnerable, however, because of those animals without a history of stress.

In view of the lesions encountered it is felt that the concept is valid and basic to the hypothesis. It has been possible to find lesions, often only histologically appreciable, in virtually every case of exhaustion shock. Four or five cases, with no gross or microscopic lesions other than those of exhaustion shock, had a history of recurrent attacks of colic. It is possible that there are no persistent lesions in such cases, or that we have not found or not recognized them.

It is felt that either prolonged exposure to a single stress (such as viral rhinitis, focal pneumonia, or myocarditis) or the addition of a new stress to an animal in the resistance phase as a result of a previous stress can precipitate the exhaustion shock phase. Note particularly that resistance to a particular stress is accompanied by decreased resistance to other stresses. In the past, horses shipped long distances by rail were off-loaded in an exhausted condition. Many, allowed to drink water before eating, died with hemorrhagic colitis. This may be considered as acute water intoxication (second stress) applied to an animal already under the effects of primary stresses of fatigue, hunger, and "emotional strain."

An example of prolonged exposure to a single stress might be that of the hemorrhagic colitis which developed in draft horses worked heavily over long periods.

The predominant localization of lesions in the large intestine in exhaustion shock requires comment. Several explanations are possible, although it is possible that none of them is completely correct.

Because shock of whatever variety causes damage throughout the circulatory system and is not restricted to any one organ or system of organs, it is not appropriate to consider the large intestine the "shock organ" of the horse. The predominant localization of overt signs of damage in the lung of the guinea pig and the liver of the dog is based on the anatomy of these particular organs (smooth muscle development). Similarly, in the horse the large intestine is a highly developed and specialized organ with an abundant vascular system. When peripheral vascular failure occurs, then, one might anticipate that the large intestine would show more striking effects than other organs.

In view of the bacterial flora of the large intestine and the high degree of fermentative and digestive activity it would be reasonable to assume that ileus, edema, and hemorrhage would, by compromising the selective absorptive ability of the epithelium, allow absorption of toxic amines, endotoxins, and the like. These products, in turn, would cause further vascular failure, perpetuating the cycle. The lesions present in the large intestine are qualitatively identical to those seen whenever the venous drainage of the intestine is blocked, as in volvulus, strangulation, or incarceration.

A relationship between exhaustion shock and intravenous tetracycline drugs has been observed. It appears that tetracycline administered to a sick animal may serve as the second stress and precipitate exhaustion shock. A specific hypersensitivity reaction in the individual animal, however, cannot be ruled out. Oxytetracycline is considered to be more toxic than the other derivatives.

There is one instance, unfortunately common, when autopsy presents difficult interpretive problems. A young horse, usually in training or at work, suddenly becomes ill with fever, muddy membranes, rapid pulse, sweating, and mild or severe diarrhea and dies quickly (within 48 hours). While these clinical signs can apply to acute salmonellosis, exhaustion shock, thrombotic or thromboembolic colic, in the case under discussion the autopsy does not reveal these conditions. There are asphyxial lesions, subcutaneous dehydration, cloudy swelling of parenchymatous organs, severe adrenal cortical hemorrhage, and splenic congestion. The contents of the large intestine are fluid and foul-smelling and there are mucosal, perhaps serosal, petechiae. The small intestine is not remarkable. There are fine erosions of the esophageal mucosa. Bacteriological studies are noncontributory; virological studies (very limited to date) have been negative. Histological findings only confirm the gross findings. There has been no evidence of toxic materials.

This condition may be the acute, fatal form of chronic diarrhea.

Chronic diarrhea is a common and

poorly understood affliction (6). Typically only one animal of any age is involved, but there have been several instances in which whole bands of young animals have been affected. The onset is usually characterized by acute, severe diarrhea and signs of shock (see above). A fatal outcome is feared. Recovery occurs in a few days, however, only to be succeeded by a persistent fecal consistency ranging from that of cow manure to watery feces. The texture of the feces fluctuates but it is never completely normal.

At autopsy one finds only a watery fluid content throughout the large intestine and, in most cases, fine linear erosions of the esophageal mucosa.

Spontaneous recovery has occurred in many cases without specific therapy other than attention to state of hydration. The condition is rarely fatal unless the animal becomes severely dehydrated.

At the present time the precise relationship and etiology of these two conditions is not known. I feel that they are one and the same and that careful study of the acute cases may yield the etiological agent for both.

Mycotic colitis and enteritis have been seen, rarely, in both foals and older horses after massive, continuous, and, one must say, unwise oral antibiotic therapy. The lesions are irregularly distributed throughout the small and large intestine and are typically massive hemorrhagic-bordered ulcerations of the mucosa with friable, yellowish necrotic debris adherent to the ulcerated area.

Occasionally, particularly in older horses, one may encounter numerous white fibrous tags on the serosal surfaces of any or all of the hollow viscera and the parietal peritoneum. They are somewhat more common on the large intestine. This is classifiable as healed peritonitis and may signify an earlier peritonitis or "damage" to the particular segment of viscus involved (such as obstipation).

Stomach

Ulcerations and irregular cornification of the esophageal portion of the stomach are common, particularly adjacent to the margo plicatus. These lesions are variable in extent and involve a few focal, numerous focal, or confluent areas. To some extent they are related to bot infestation (*Gasterophilus intestinalis*) or ingestion of sharp foreign material, but their precise significance and cause in any given case may be difficult to determine. Occasionally such ulcers may perforate, causing fatal peritonitis (82). Fundic ulceration has been seen in young animals severely ill and/or under heavy antibiotic and steroid therapy for protracted periods (82).

The fundic mucosa is normally pink-gray, slimy, and cobblestoned in character. All degrees of pink-red coloration may be encountered, uniformly or patchily distributed. A quantity of clear, viscid mucus is normally present.

Gastritis is uncommon in the horse, and a reddish color is not sufficient reason for the diagnosis. A true acute gastritis will be characterized by excessive mucus production, severe hyperemia, and petechiation of the mucosa. Such lesions are seen with severe *Trichostrongyle* infestation, for example.

Chronic gastritis is characterized by patchy reddening, marked increase in the coarseness of the cobblestoning, and frank nodular formations. Nodules of considerable size with apical holes are caused by *Draschia megastoma*. *Habronema* infestation may be sufficiently severe to cause chronic gastritis involving all or a portion of the fundic mucosa. Some cases of chronic gastritis, in older horses, are of unknown etiology (16).

G. nasalis may be found in considerable numbers in the pylorus and first part of the duodenum, usually without evidence of inflammation. Blackish discoloration of the mucosa is not uncommon as a postmortem phenomenon (H_2S).

Carcinoma of the stomach has been reported in horses (squamous cell carcinoma of the esophageal and adenocarcinoma of the fundic region (53)), but I have not seen a case.

Small Intestine

As a rule only small amounts of ingesta are in the small intestine. The mucosa is normally grayish-tan in color with a considerable quantity of clear, watery mucus in the lumen and clinging to the mucosal surface. Enteritis is exceedingly rare in my experience. *Shigella* and *E. coli* septicemias in foals, however, are frequently accompanied by a severe hemorrhagic enteritis. I have seen only one bona fide case of acute catarrhal enteritis in an adult horse; the cause of the enteritis was not determined by histology, bacteriology, or virology.

Parasitic lesions are common. Solitary nodules bulge into the lumen from the submucosa. They may have apical orifices, and gentle pressure or incision frees a caseous or purulent content. These are reactions to strongyle larvae entrapped in the gut wall.

The ileum is normally thicker and more hose-like than the jejunum. Strongyle migration lesions are common (31–34) (see Chapter 2). In fact, *S. vulgaris* appears to preferentially enter the circulatory system in the ileum. The acute migration lesion is severe greenish edema and some hemorrhage in the submucosa, muscularis, and

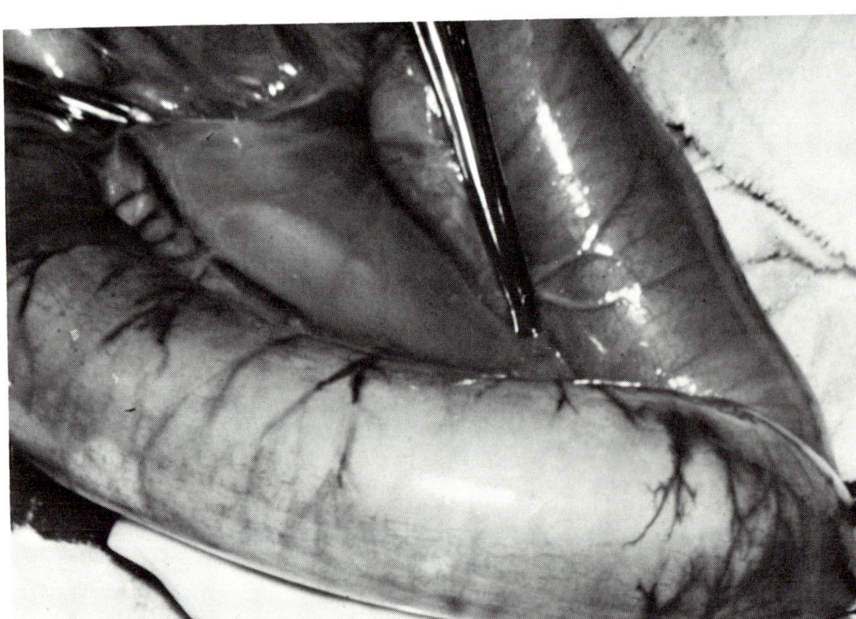

FIG. 66. Acute hemamelasma ilei. The wall of the small intestine is infarcted and hemolyzed blood is diffusing into the greenish, edematous wall (surgical photograph). This is an extreme example.

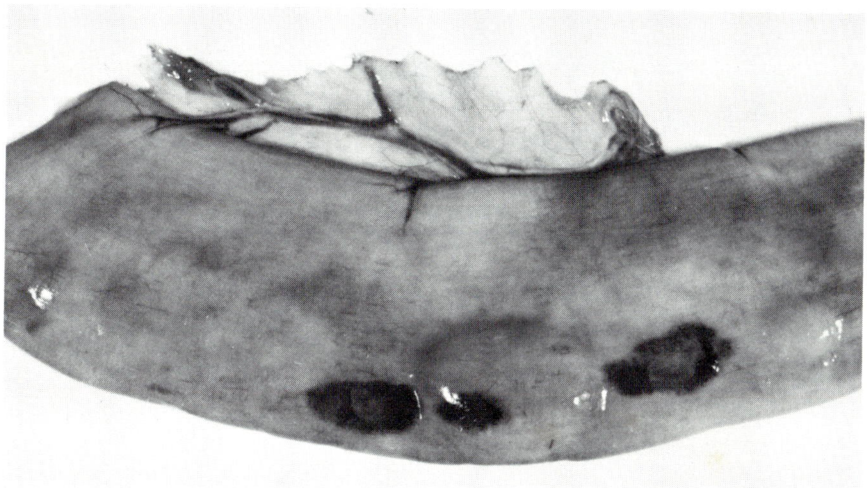

FIG. 67. Chronic hemamelasma ilei.

serosa (Fig. 66). In the more commonly observed chronic lesion there is an elevated fibrous plaque on the serosa, which is greenish-black and/or hemorrhagic (hemamelasma ilei) (Fig. 67). Occasionally, ridgelike blackish elevations of the mucosa are the only lesions, and (rarely) there may be both serosal and mucosal involvement. Sufficiently severe larval migration in the wall of ileum may cause massive submucosal fibrosis and compensatory muscular hyperplasia.

Anoplocephala magna may be encountered in small numbers in the small intestine.

Occasionally, in a young horse with a history of recurrent, low-grade, obstipation-type colic, autopsy reveals a thickened rigid ileum with infiltration of white masses in the submucosa and mucosa. This is lymphosarcoma.

I have seen three or four cases of thickening of the ileum and regional lymph nodes which appeared grossly to be lymphosarcoma. Microscopically, however, there was a severe granulomatous process with fibrosis, macrophages, and giant cells. No organisms could be detected with bacterial, acid-fast, or fungal stains, and cultural attempts were not satisfactory (no attempt was made to isolate acid-fast or fungal organisms). It has been noted, however (50), that the tubercle organism may be difficult to detect. I have not seen pulmonary or generalized tuberculosis in the horse (68).

Colic

Malpositions, infarctions and "colics" are frequent problems in horses. In what follows I shall attempt to present a reasonable hypothesis for these several conditions, emphasizing basic similarities.

Whenever a malposition is encountered, the prosector should determine precisely what elements are involved, how they are twisted or entrapped, where they are located, and to what extent the part is involved. If possible, correction of the malposition *in situ* will permit determination of all these factors. Often, because of the degree of involvement or postmortem changes (friable intestine), it is not possible to physically reposition the gut *in situ*.

Causes

Acute
- Ligature
- Lipoma
- Herniation
- anoxia, acute
  - A. Verminous thrombosis
  - B. Other
- Inflammation
  - A. Larval migration
  - B. Other
- Gaseous feed
- Neural reflex inhibition (sympathetic discharge causes anoxia by vasoconstriction—gastritis, postoperative peritonitis, pain of other origin)

Chronic
- Ulceration-stricture
- Dry feed
- Herniation
- Anoxia, chronic
  - A. Worms
  - B. Other

↓

Segmental Ileus

Results

Fast
- Intussusception
- Strangulation
- Incarceration
- Volvulus
- *Strongylus vulgaris*
  - A. Thrombotic
  - B. Thromboembolic

Slow
- Musculofibrous hyperplasia (proximal to lesion)

FIG. 68. Segmental ileus hypothesis. See text for details.

The repositioning must, then, be accomplished by palpation and intellectual effort on the part of the prosector. Particular attention must be paid to lesions other than the obvious malposition in the search for proximate causes of the malposition. I should like to present the hypothesis summarized in Figure 68, as an explanation for the cause of malposition and many other gastrointestinal problems of horses. Basic and central to this hypothesis is segmental ileus, i.e., a portion of the intestine stops moving while the remainder of the intestine continues to move (81). If a bolus of potentially gaseous food material is moving down the small intestine and slows down between peristaltic waves, sufficient gas may be produced to mechanically, or by toxic action, partially or completely inhibit muscular activity in the immediate vicinity. Similarly, if an embolus blocks an arterial branch to a segment of intestine, there may be either temporary or permanent anoxia of the intestinal segment. Acute anoxia is a clear cause of segmental ileus. Chronic or (better, perhaps) partial anoxia is not quite as clear-cut and is discussed in greater detail below. The possible role of anatomical lesions of neural elements as the cause of segmental ileus is problematical. I have not been able to directly or with reasonable certainty indirectly incriminate autonomic dysfunction as a cause of segmental ileus, as attractive as the possibilities are. The various facets of the hypothesis will be brought out in more detail as we consider the individual gastrointestinal lesions which cause or can cause fatal "colic".

Strongylus vulgaris. First, we shall consider the effects of *S. vulgaris* (94) larval thrombosis of the ileocecocolic artery. There are two distinct pathological entities, which may be called thrombotic and thromboembolic infarction.

In the thrombotic form the clinical

course is fulminant with severe shock, dehydration, and early death—identical to the clinical signs of exhaustion shock. At autopsy the cecum and ventral and dorsal colon are diffusely muddy-red and filled with liquid and/or blood-tinged ingesta. The ileocecocolic artery is firmly plugged with a friable, brownish mass of fibrin containing immature larvae. It is my impression that the blood supply to the cecum and dorsal and ventral colon has been totally obstructed as a single event in a short period of time. Ileus, shock, and death supervene before gross morphological evidence of ischemic necrosis of the bowel wall can occur.

In the second, classic thromboembolic form (Fig. 69) the clinical course may be somewhat more prolonged and relapsing in nature. At autopsy, frank segmental necrosis and gangrene of the large intestine is found associated with multiple emboli in the related vessels. The thrombus in the ileocecocolic artery may be small, although obviously it is small because of the multiple emboli which have broken off and moved down the branches of the ileocecocolic artery. Thrombi in this artery tend to be either sessile, with less chance of embolization, or pedunculated and tear-drop shaped, with a greater risk of embolization.

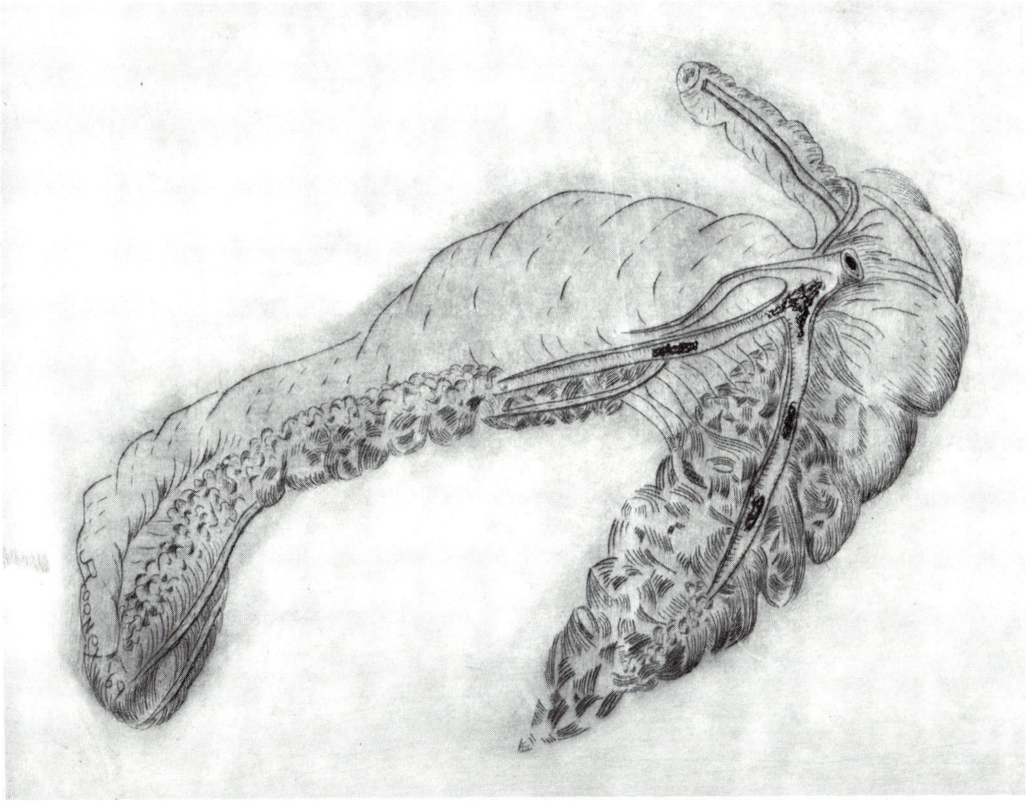

FIG. 69. Thromboemobolic disease of the large intestine. Thrombus in the ileocecocolic artery with emboli in the medial cecal and ventral colic artery. Infarction of the cecum and ventral colon. (Dry point etching.)

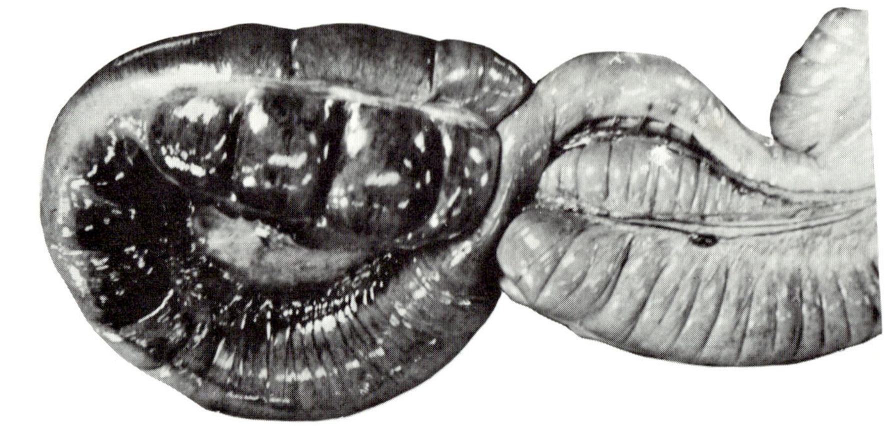

FIG. 70. Torsion of the colon at the sternal-diaphragmatic flexures. There were parasitic emboli in the dorsal and ventral colic arteries at the flexures.

Emboli may cause torsion of the colon (see Chapter 2) (Fig. 70) as well as the classic thromboembolic infarction, and it is important, particularly for the beginner, to make a habit of routinely opening all the branches of the cranial mesenteric artery.

There is yet a third type of infarction to be considered. Occasionally a horse may acquire a massive infestation of *S. vulgaris* larvae either experimentally or by grazing a heavily infested pasturage (race horses grassed around stables, for example). In such cases the flood of larvae migrating in the jejunal arteries can cause infarction of one or more segments of the jejunum, usually the middle or lower third, or the ileum (Fig. 65). While this condition is uncommon it should be looked for, and the affected segment of gut and mesenteric vessels should be carefully examined, under magnification, for immature larvae.

In all these types of *S. vulgaris* damage, vascular blockage, anoxia, and, inevitably, segmental ileus are the significant factors. In thrombotic colic, for example, there is ileus of the entire large intestine. With thromboembolism there is segmental ileus carried to the logical extreme of total necrosis.

Acute gastric dilatation and rupture. Rupture is a simple matter. The peritoneal cavity is full of ingesta. As is well known the rupture occurs along the greater curvature, and the tear is most extensive in the serosa, somewhat less extensive in the muscularis, and least extensive in the mucosa which bulges or pouts outward. Such rupture may be expected as soon as the abdomen is opened because of packing of ingesta in and around the greater omentum (Fig. 71).

Acute gastric dilatation without rupture can be a difficult postmortem diagnosis. Postmortem gaseous distension of the stomach is routine and the diagnosis cannot be made on that factor alone. In some cases, at least, slight or moderate tearing of the serosa may be apparent together with petechiae or small extravasations of blood on the greater curvature of the stomach. These findings, together with an appropriate history, make the diagnosis firm. An animal may develop acute gastric dilatation during the night and die before morning. Careful study of the greater curvature of the stomach as indicated above may permit at least a probable diagnosis of acute gastric dilatation.

In established or tentative cases of acute

gastric dilatation the duodenum should be carefully examined. Frank strictures or stenoses of the duodenum are an obvious anatomical cause for the dilatation. In so-called idiopathic cases there may well be an ileus of the duodenum. As indicated in Figure 16, the descending limb of the duodenum has both a vascular and neural end-to-end arrangement without the regular segmental vascularization and innervation of the remainder of the small intestine (see, however, *Strangulation*, below). It is reasonable, then, to suggest that temporary ileus of this segment of the duodenum may be caused by any of the functional factors shown in Figure 68. Such a segment of intestine will be more susceptible to anoxia because of the vascular pattern.

Volvulus. Volvulus is a twisting of the small intestine around the mesenteric axis. It presents readily and startlingly when the abdomen is opened. The corkscrew coils of distended, dark-red small intestine bulge upward immediately (Fig. 72). To reduce the volvulus *in situ* it may be necessary to decompress each loop. The twisting may be in either direction and be 180° or more. The distal extent, in my experience, has always been the ileum. The proximal limit is variable but never farther, of course, than the duodenocolic ligament (anatomical junction of ascending limb of duodenum and jejunum).

One must carefully evaluate all blood vessels and the ingesta in an attempt to define the cause of the volvulus. According to the hypothesis presented, segmental ileus, with or without hyperperistalsis, is the cause, and the search must be for the cause of the segmental ileus. An analogy may help to clarify the role of such ileus (Fig. 73). When the rope is grasped (ileus), the traveling wave will wrap around the hand. In the case of the small intestine the "dead" segment is not a fixed axis and the intestine will wrap around the fixed axis, the root of the mesentery.

It is noteworthy that the autopsy incidence of volvulus (as well as strangulation, incarceration, and intussusception)

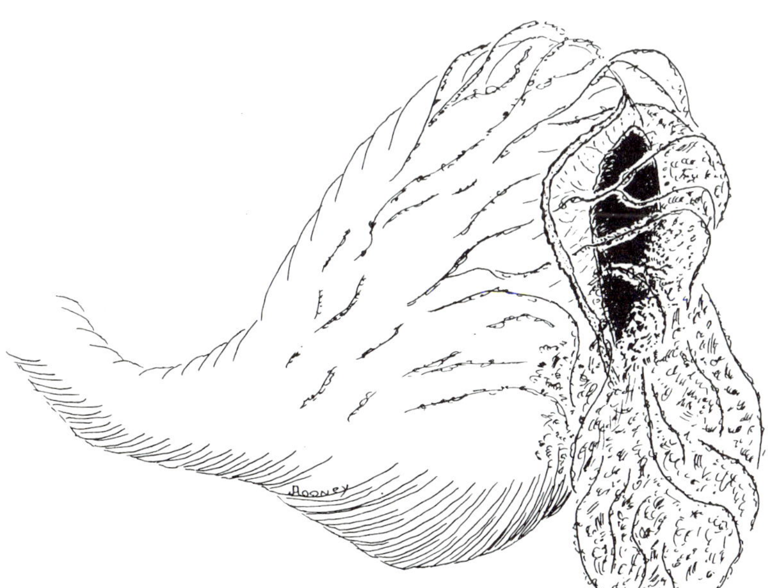

FIG. 71. Rupture of the stomach with ingesta spilling into and distending the greater omentum.

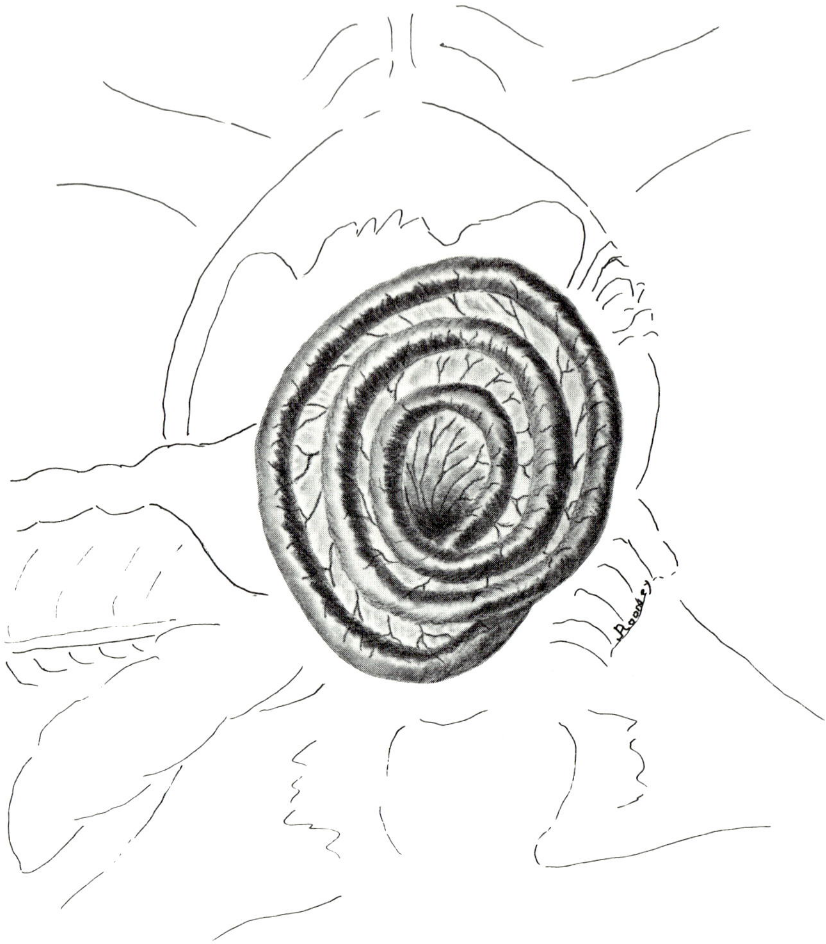

FIG. 72. Volvulus of the small intestine.

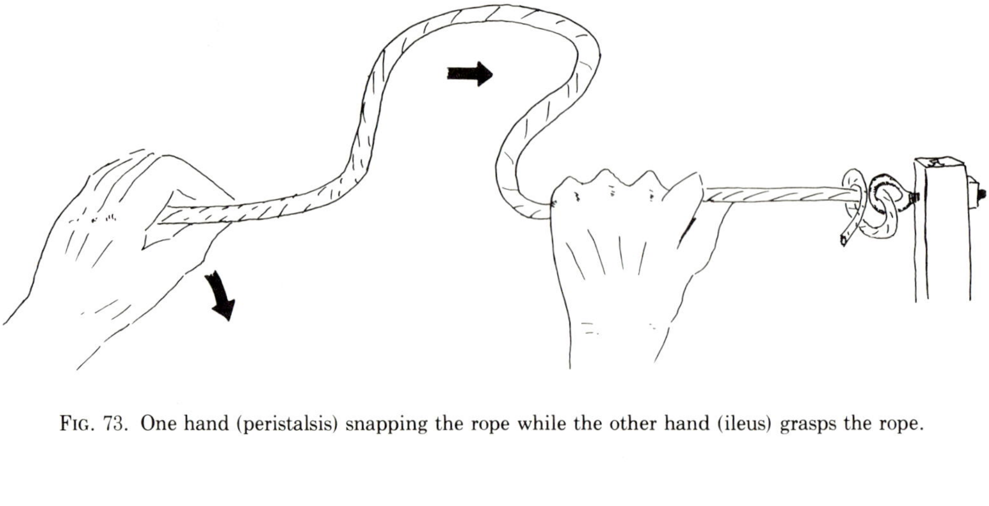

FIG. 73. One hand (peristalsis) snapping the rope while the other hand (ileus) grasps the rope.

had declined precipitously with the establishment of thorough, regular worming programs. It is my feeling, therefore, that the most common cause of segmental ileus in the horse is the anoxia and/or inflammation caused by *Strongylus* spp. migrations. In a given case it may be difficult to identify the microscopic larvae traveling in vessels of the small intestine, causing temporary anoxia. When a young horse is exposed either experimentally or inadvertently to a massive dose of strongyle larvae, however, the numbers of microscopic larvae invading the small intestine and traversing the mesenteric vessels may be so great that infarction of segments of the small intestine occurs (Fig. 74). If such massive blockage of vessels by larvae traveling toward the cranial mesenteric artery can occur, it is reasonable that smaller numbers may produce a temporary blockage or, at least, a compromising of the circulation with temporary anoxia. Further, it appears from autopsy experience that strongyle larvae invade in greatest numbers through the terminal portion of the jejunum and the ileum. (Further evidence for this is discussed in connection with intussusception.) This correlates well with the predilection of the ileum for segmental ileus; volvulus, incarceration, strangulation, and the like are most common in or near the ileum.

Strangulation. Strangulation occurs when a loop of intestine ties a knot in itself without rupturing the mesentery. The site of the tying may vary but appears to be most common close to the ileocecal junction. The lesion may not be immediately apparent when the abdomen is opened (at autopsy or time of surgery), but the small intestine will be markedly distended proximal to the lesion, suggesting immediate examination of the ileum.

The anatomical arrangement of the

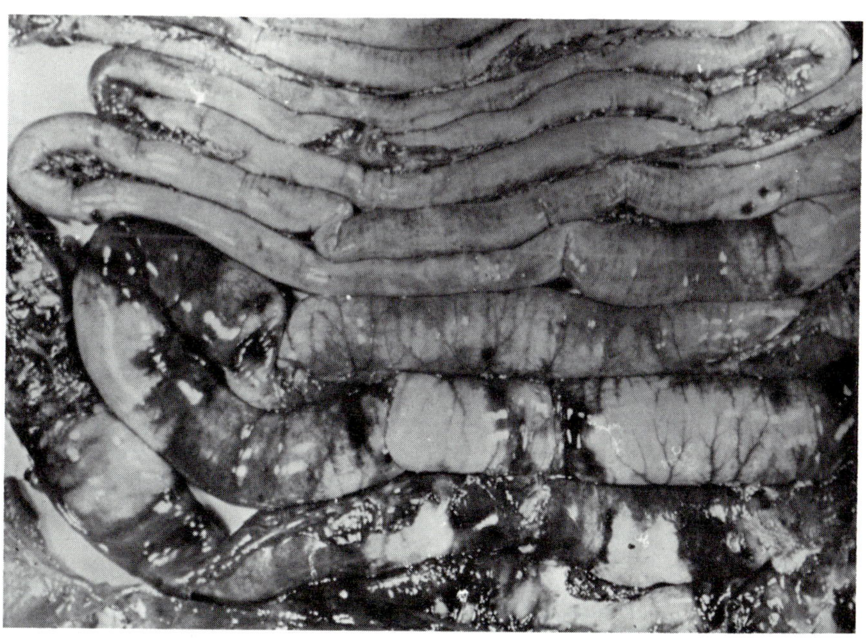

FIG. 74. Infarction of the small intestine by massive *Strongylus vulgaris* invasion. Normal above and infarcted below.

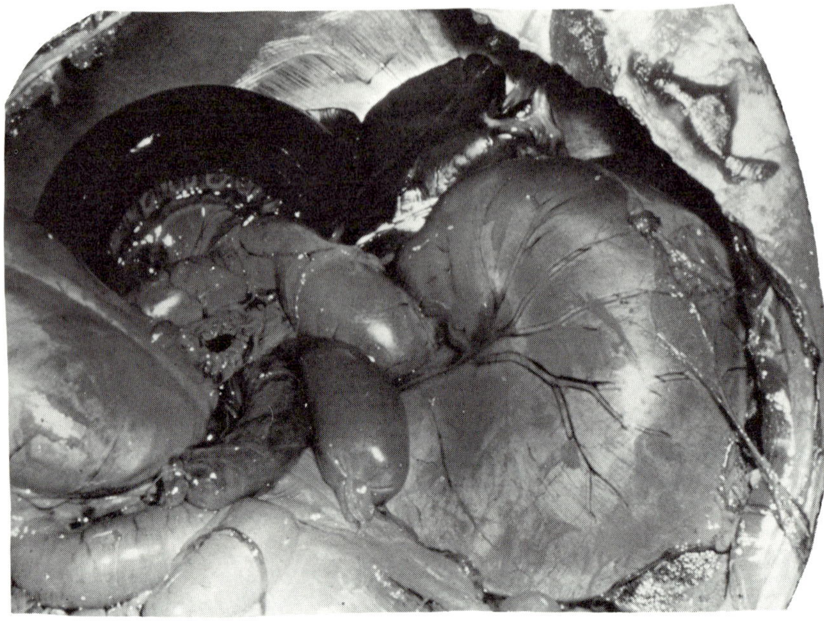

FIG. 75. Incarceration of the small intestine through the epiploic foramen. From the two tied-off ends the jejunum passes under (dorsal to) the duodenum to form the dark, distended loop. The transverse colon has been displaced to the right.

vessels and nerves of the ileum is similar to that of the duodenum (Fig. 8) and immediately suggests that this segment of the intestine should be peculiarly sensitive to vascular blockage. In addition, the work of Alexander (3) indicates that the ileum is particularly sensitive to anoxia, at least in the isolated state.

Incarceration. Incarceration is similar to strangulation. A loop of jejunum bursts through the mesentery and becomes entrapped. Once again, this lesion occurs most frequently near the ileocecal junction. The intestine may rupture the mesentery and entrap as a single event. In some cases the defect in the mesentery is obviously older than the incarceration (the edges of the hole are rounded, smooth, and firm), suggesting that the rupture occurred some time earlier and the intestine retreated before it became entrapped in the mesenteric defect it had produced. Occasionally, a rent may be found in the mesentery as an incidental autopsy finding. In addition to being a threat for eventual incarceration the presence of such rents supports the above suggestion that rents can occur without the intestine becoming permanently entrapped at the time it bursts through the mesentery.

Special Incarcerations. Special cases of incarceration are seen infrequently. Epiploic foramen incarceration may be suspected as soon as the abdomen is opened by the position of a loop of dark-red distended intestine on the right side between the right lobe of the liver and the duodenum (Fig. 75). Epiploic incarcerations are usually seen in older horses and may or may not be related to atrophy of a lobe of the liver.

I have seen only three cases of incarceration in the gastrosplenic ligament. In two a loop of small intestine had incarcerated, and in one the pelvic flexure of the colon had passed through an old, smooth-edged rent.

Incarceration of a loop of small intestine by a pedunculated lipoma is not uncommon in older horses (Fig. 76). With increasing age lipomas of the mesentery become more and more frequent. If such fatty masses achieve sufficient size and/or undergo necrosis and calcification, they become pedunculated, and one can envision them snaking about in the peritoneal cavity like a lethal bolo. It is only a matter of time and chance until a loop of small intestine is tied by a half hitch of the thin, rope-like pedicle of the lipoma.

Diaphragmatic Hernia. Diaphragmatic hernia may be included in this discussion since a fatal outcome is invariably due to incarceration of either the small or large intestine. There are three types of diaphragmatic hernia. The first occurs near the xiphoid cartilage (midline, ventral) and is purely and solely a postmortem rupture of the diaphragm.

The second and third types are both rare. The second is a smooth-edged defect in the left dorsal aspect of the diaphragm, which appears to be congenital in origin. The third, apparently a traumatic form, may involve any part of the diaphragm but most often involves the left middle portion. I have never seen a diaphragmatic defect, congenital or traumatic, in the right half of the diaphragm.

Intussusception. Intussusception of the small intestine is most common in suckling foals. It may occur at any point

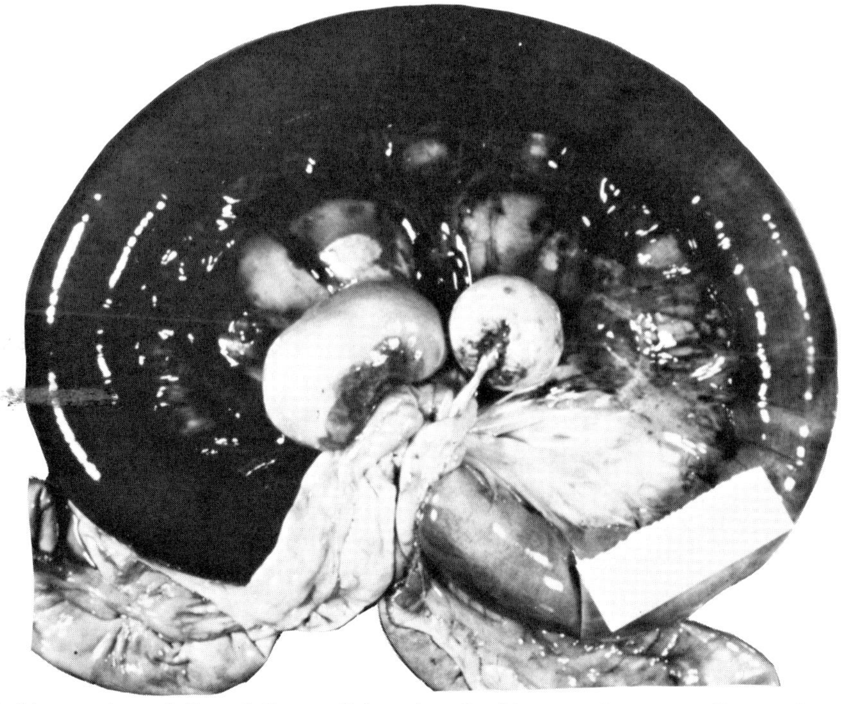

FIG. 76. Lipoma strangulation of the small intestine. In this unusual case two lipomas have tied half-hitches around the intestine.

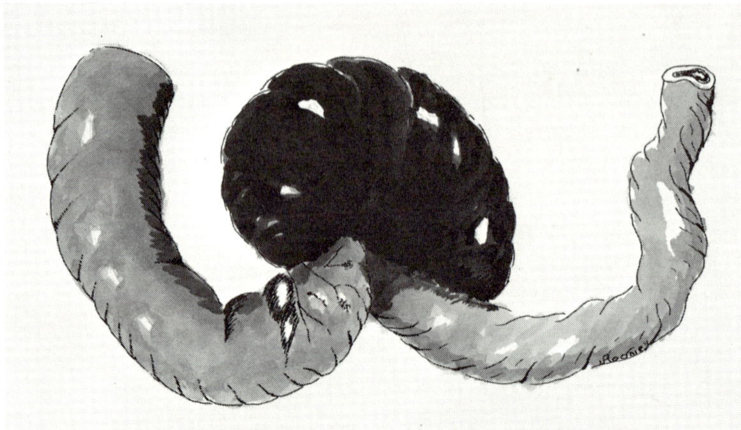

FIG. 77. Double intussusception of the jejunum of a foal.

in the jejunum, may be multiple, or may even have a second intussusception superimposed upon the primary intussusception (Fig. 77). These latter cases are clear examples of segmental ileus (the first intussusception) resulting in intestinal malposition (the second intussusception). The cause of the first intussusception, however, has in my experience never been clear. One may glibly speak of an immature neural controlling mechanism and aberrant eating habits; both are undoubtedly factors, but they are difficult to document on morphological grounds. Segmental ileus must occur, but the precise cause of the ileus is unknown in most cases. Parasitic activity has not been apparent in most cases, although strongyle migration and/or ascarid infestation have been present in a few cases.

Agonal intussusception is common in foals and readily differentiated because of the lack of marked vascular stasis. Some agonal intussusceptions, however, may have a moderate degree of hyperemia (depending, obviously, on how long they were present before death), and the prosector should not be satisfied with such a lesion unless no other lesions are apparent or the history is compatible (severe abdominal pain and early profound shock causing death before marked stasis develops).

Intussusception in older horses is uncommon in my experience and has invariably been intussusception of the ileum into the cecum. In all of my cases there has been significant acute or chronic (Figs. 66 and 67) parasitic involvement of the ileum. These hemamelasma ilei provide the segmental ileus necessary for intussusception to occur. A peristaltic wave (in fact the neural and/or myogenic controlling pattern of the wave) is disrupted, causing the wave to overrun and result in an intussusception.

Colon Rotation. Rotation of the colon classically (16) involves a twist of 90° or more of the large intestine localized at the diaphragmatic-sternal flexures. The left dorsal and ventral portions of the colon are involved. An ingenious mechanical explanation has been offered (27). The few cases that I have seen, however, have always been associated with verminous emboli in the dorsal and ventral colic arteries (Fig. 70). Acute ischemia (anoxia) may, then, be incriminated as the immediate cause of the segmental ileus leading to torsion by way of the suggested mechanical pathway.

In recent years there has been an apparent increase in the incidence of torsion of the entire dorsal and ventral colon. The site of the twist is at the origin of the ventral colon and termination of the dorsal colon, the cecum and descending colon not being involved. Most cases have been in older horses. In all cases there has been atrophy of the right lobe of the liver which could be interpreted as providing "dead space" for rotation to occur. This hypothesis, however, is not very attractive. Pressure by the colon on the right lobe is suggested as the cause of the atrophy, and it is reasonable, therefore, that the colon would occupy the space as soon as the liver disappears, leaving no dead space. I have no explanation for such torsions. Since all other forms of malpositioning appear to be related to segmental ileus, I see no reason to make an exception in this particular case. To date, however, I have not been able to find any direct evidence of ileus in this type of colon rotation.

I would like to digress at this point to lay an old ghost. In the absence of other explanations, rolling of the horse has been suggested as a cause of gut twists. This action has no significance, except perhaps with colon torsions. The horse would have to spin on his back like a dervish to cause a volvulus, for example.

Rupture of Cecum and Rectum. During the immediate postpartum period clinical signs of severe peritonitis may appear. At autopsy such cases are frequently found to be the result of rupture of the cecum or rectum. In the latter case the site of rupture may be suspected immediately by the packing of masses of ingesta in the pelvic area. In cecal rupture no such distinct localization is apparent. Whereas the rectum ruptures on the ventral surface, the cecum ruptures in the middle third of the medial surface (Fig. 78) and may be easily overlooked unless the cecocolic ligament is severed and the cecum separated from the right ventral colon.

The cause of these two ruptures is not definitely known, but it appears reasonable that the extreme pressure of the parturition process, particularly with a large foal, could burst the rectum like a balloon. Similarly, if the cecum retroflexes with the apex extending into the pelvic cavity, the outrushing foal may rupture the cecum like a balloon. Since it is known that the cecum can occasionally retroflex in this manner, the hypothesis has some strength.

Nonparturient rectal ruptures in mares as well as in foals with meconium impaction hardly require comment. The major problem of the pathologist is how to report such ruptures.

Postoperative Ileus. There are many facets to the developing subject of equine abdominal surgery, and I intend to cover only that one portion directly related to pathology. Obviously, many unsuccessful surgical cases are directly related to delay

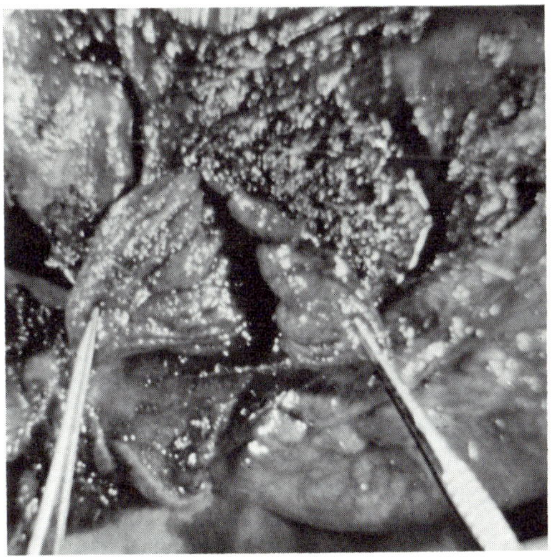

FIG. 78. Rupture of the cecum.

in deciding that surgery should be done—that is, when shock, toxemia, and general debilitation have proceeded too far for the animal to be able to withstand the additional stress of anesthesia and major surgery.

Unfortunately, a large number of horses subjected to technically successful abdominal surgery succumb at some variable time postoperatively. The postoperative clinical course usually includes variably severe abdominal pain and distension. The animal may live for a week or more with variable degrees of colicky pain, only to succumb in the end to acute gastric dilatation and rupture despite the fact that the original lesion had been adequately and completely repaired.

The autopsy in such cases may be morphologically disappointing at first glance. If the autopsy is performed shortly after death, the small intestine may be distended with gas, and it is reasonable to suggest that postoperative ileus was the basic pathophysiological problem. The precise nature of postoperative ileus has not been divined, but it may be suggested that painful stimuli initiate a sympathetic (splanchnic) discharge which inhibits gut motility.

Chronic Colic. The classical example of chronic colic is chronic typhlitis (16, 23). The muscularis and submucosa of the cecum are greatly increased in thickness, converting the cecal wall to a tough, leathery consistency. There may be multiple small fibrous tags on the serosal surface.

While the cecum is the classically described case, such changes may be found in localized segments of the ventral colon, the transverse colon, jejunum, and ileum (85). There is invariably muscular hypertrophy and hyperplasia, and there may or may not be submucosal fibrosis.

The clinical course is characterized by low-grade, recurrent colic of considerable duration—months to years. To date, there has been no clinical differentiation of the site of the primary lesion, and it is unlikely that such differentiation could be achieved with present techniques. A fatal outcome, in the absence of surgery, has invariably been the result of rupture of the bowel at some point proximal to the area of musculofibrous hyperplasia.

The precise cause of this type of lesion is speculative, but the following observations may be offered. (1) In a few cases, careful dissection of the vessels has uncovered one or more parasitic emboli in small vessels in or near the area of musculofibrous hyperplasia. (2) If a segment of intestine is incompletely obstructed by a chronic ulcer or adhesion (postoperative, *C. equi* abscess, or a variety of undetermined), the intestine for a variable distance above the site of the obstruction will show musculofibrous hyperplasia. It may be suggested, then, that this lesion results from segmental ileus—what one might call a "slow" ileus as opposed to the fast, acute type which leads to volvulus, incarceration, etc. (Fig. 68). The gradual stricture development would impede the movement of ingesta and result in hyperplasia; the muscle thickens in an attempt to push ingesta past the stricture. Parasitic emboli, causing partial anoxia and ischemia, may devitalize a segment of intestine sufficiently to inhibit or stop muscular activity but not be severe enough to cause necrosis and gangrene. Musculofibrous hyperplasia may then occur just proximal to the area of ileus.

There is some support for this hypothesis. Experimental infection of worm-free ponies with *S. edentatus* is accompanied by severe thrombosis and fibrosis of the neurovascular complexes of the cecum. As a result, severe musculofibrous hyperplasia of the cecal wall occurs. It presently appears that the massive fibrosis and thrombosis of the cecal vessels is caused by migration of *S. edentatus* larvae. The specimens I have seen have been so severely involved that a clear distinction could not be made as to the primary vessel of involvement (artery or vein); the impression is that the vein is primarily involved.

Rider (89, 90) described a form of chronic musculofibrous hyperplasia, sometimes associated with macroscopic diverticula, in the small intestine of pit ponies. The cause was not determined.

Nonfatal Colic. Finally, we shall take up the question of nonfatal colic. It is true that as regular egg counts and worming routines are established in a band of horses the incidence of colic signs decreases markedly. This point cannot be emphasized too strongly. There is a near linear relationship between the incidence of both fatal and nonfatal colic and the adequacy of the worm control program. The basic answer to colic in horses does not lie in the development of improved medical or surgical procedures; it lies in the control of worms. This is unglamorous, perhaps, but it is a simple, bald fact.

It has been suggested (67) that the inflammatory reaction incited by bloodworm larvae in the ileocecocolic artery involves the cranial mesenteric ganglion and the autonomic nerves issuing from that ganglion. My observations indicate that the ganglion cells and nerve fibers are singularly resistant to damage. Indeed, nerve bundles can be seen, microscopically, passing unscathed through areas of massive fibrosis and chronic inflammatory reaction. Hirose and Satoh's elaborate study (41), developing an "autonomic-neurogenic theory," unfortunately shows only normal and postmortem phenomena.

It appears more reasonable that the nonfatal colics related to worm infestation are caused by larval migrations and the intravascular thrombosing processes which accompany such migrations. Larvae migrating in vessels can cause transitory ischemia of the intestinal wall supplied by such vessels. Ischemia causes ileus. Segmental ileus can prevent the passage of ingesta and/or gas, in turn leading to distension of the intestine and pain. The inflammatory reaction which inevitably accompanies larval penetration of the mucosa and submucosa of the gut may well initiate painful sensory discharges. Such sensory discharges initiate sympathetic motor activity through the splanchnic nerves which, in turn, cause constriction of blood vessels, ischemia, and consequently ileus.

This is a reasonable interpretation based on the study of fatal colics at autopsy. If segmental ileus can result in volvulus, strangulation, and intussusception, it is reasonable that lesser degrees of ileus or ileus of a transitory nature could cause the temporary stoppages, gaseous distension, cramping, and pain characteristic of most nonfatal colics. In other words, it is suggested that fatal colic and nonfatal colic are simply different degrees of the same basic process. Ileus can be measured on several scales to correspond with the degrees of clinical severity of the colic process. The ileus may be of shorter or longer duration and of varying intensity—complete or partial ileus, complete stoppage, or simply slowing.

Following the same line of reasoning, massive, severe verminous infestation is not necessary to cause colic. Heavy infestation, for example, may cause thrombotic or thromboembolic colic whereas lesser degrees of infestation may lead to strangulation or incarceration. At the lower, or "least," end of the scale are the temporary stoppages of nonfatal colic.

I think the reader can immediately accept that *S. vulgaris* is not the only cause of colic, as is indicated in Figure 68. The important point, the unifying general case, is segmental ileus. In the horse, at least, *S. vulgaris* is simply the most common special case.

Irvine (44) has delineated a syndrome, protein-losing enteropathy, in which "...a change occurs in the gut wall which allows transudation into the gut lumen of protein molecules, mainly of small size, such as albumin. As the ability of the sole albumin-forming organ, the liver, to increase albumin production is rather limited, hypoalbuminemia is a common result. Clinically, this appears as protein-wasting malnutrition and, when serum albumin drops to about 2 Gm. %, edema. Symptoms are referable also to the basic cause of disturbance, usually parasitic thrombosis, and the digestive disturbance which accompanies it, for example, recurrent colic.

"In differential diagnosis, one must consider the other causes of hypoalbuminemia, which can be grouped into (a) inadequate formation and (b) excessive degradation. In the first group, general nutritional errors, malabsorption and hypermotility will decrease the availability of albumin precursors, and are readily identifiable. Because almost all albumin synthesis occurs in the liver, any disturbance of this organ may cause hypoalbuminemia. While this is not common, its presence is determinable by a battery of liver function tests. Excessively rapid degradation may result from albumin leakage, or from hypercatabolism in tissue. Of the former, the only real possibility, apart from obvious accidents such as shock, crush or burns, is albuminuria, and this may be readily checked. Of the hypercatabolic causes, febrile conditions, exercise to excess, and the hypermetabolic conditions, are possibilities."

Although this syndrome cannot be diagnosed by postmortem pathological techniques, it should be kept in mind, particularly when the prosector is confronted with a case of idiopathic cachexia and inanition.

NINE

The Pharynx, Larynx, and Heart

Dissection

Open the dorsal wall of the pharynx, continuing the incision through the esophagus. Examine the lingual, palatine, and pharyngeal mucosa and tonsillar tissue. Examine and slice the thyroids. Locate and examine the parathyroid glands. The internal glands are embedded in fat in the vicinity of the cranial thyroid artery. The external glands are along the ventral surface of the trachea often as far caudally as the carotid bifurcation.

Slice and examine the tongue. Strip the esophagus forward to the pharyngeal orifice, exposing the dorsal surface of the larynx.

Examine the extrinsic and intrinsic muscles of the larynx (Fig. 79). The cricoarytenoideus lateralis, ventricularis, and vocalis muscles are exposed by cutting away the lamina of the thyroid cartilage. Open the larynx on the dorsal midline and examine the folds and saccules.

The heart and lungs will be dissected together to maintain the proper anatomical relationships. They will be separated when those relationships have been completely explored. Although the dissection is somewhat more difficult to learn, the advantages of maintaining precise anatomical relationships far outweigh the initial technical difficulties. The blood flow method is not used since, as will be seen, the more ventrally placed pulmonary veins must be opened and examined before the pulmonary artery.

Separate the aorta from the mediastinum, leaving it attached at the base of the heart. Free the esophagus from the mediastinum. This is most readily accomplished by blunt dissection. Minimal sharp dissection may be necessary over the base of the heart. Open the esophagus. Slice and examine the thymus, if present. It is usually completely (grossly) atrophied by one year of age.

Turn the heart and lungs upside down so that the ventral surfaces of the lungs are uppermost and the trachea (tongue in the foal) is to the prosector's left. The left lateral surface of the heart is presented for examination by drawing the apex of the heart toward the prosector.

Slice the pleural connection between the middle and left lobes of the lung, continuing the incision to the left, opening the pericardium (Fig. 80). Open the pericardium to the apex of the heart, noting the amount, color, and content of the pericardial fluid. Do not attempt to remove the pericardium completely at this stage.

With the knife, open the left atrium, starting at the cranial border and carrying the incision caudad out the major pulmonary veins into the lungs (Fig. 81). Remove the blood by hand wiping and examine the veins.

Palpate the left atrioventricular orifice through the atrial incision. Direct the knife through the atrium and orifice to the apex of the left ventricle close to the caudal border of the heart—the right longitudinal groove. Cut out, opening the ventricle. Examine the left atrio-ventricular (A-V) valves, chordae tendinae, endocardium, and papillary muscles (Fig. 81). They will be considered in more detail later.

In order to examine the right side of the heart, simply spin the entire specimen around so that the trachea is pointing to the right with the ventral surfaces of the lungs still uppermost (Fig.

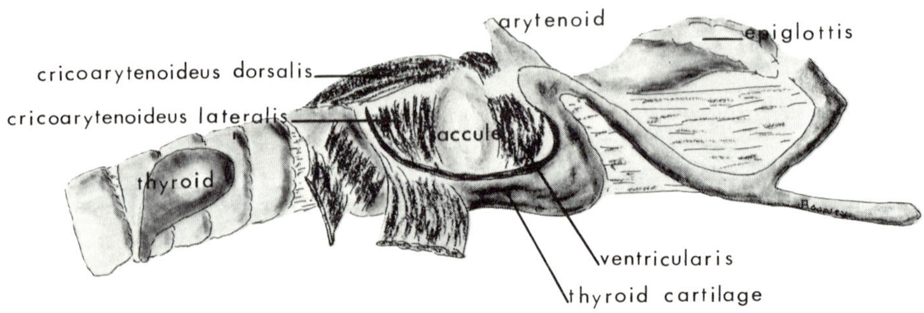

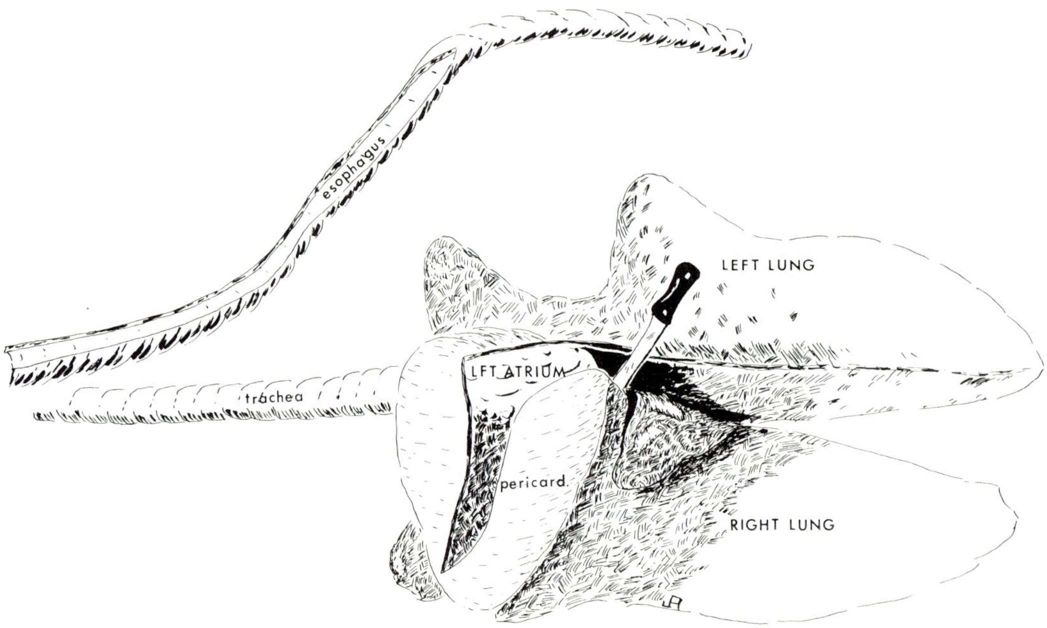

FIG. 80. The lungs are upside down and the trachea is to the prosector's left. The left side of the heart is presenting with the pericardium opened and the knife separating the middle lobe of the right lung from the left lung. The esophagus was separated earlier and is shown partially opened.

82). Do not pick up the specimen to turn it or relationships will be lost. The apex of the heart is drawn toward the prosector, presenting the right lateral surface of the heart for examination. The pericardium may now be removed completely.

Open the right atrium, continuing the incision caudally to open the coronary sinus, caudodorsally to open the caudal vena cava and craniodorsally to open the cranial vena cava (Fig. 82).

Locate the foramen ovale, or its scar, and check the patency with probe or finger. Determine the patency and condition of the right atrioventricular orifice by inserting a finger through the atrium into the ventricle. Direct the knife through the caudal part of the atrium, parallel to the right longitudinal groove, to the apex of the right ventricle, and cut. Redirect the knife from the apex parallel and close to the left longitudinal groove toward the origin of the pulmonary artery and cut. Tip the apex of the heart away from the prosector. The origin and course of the pulmonary artery are now clearly displayed. Continue the cut in the right ventricle into the pul-

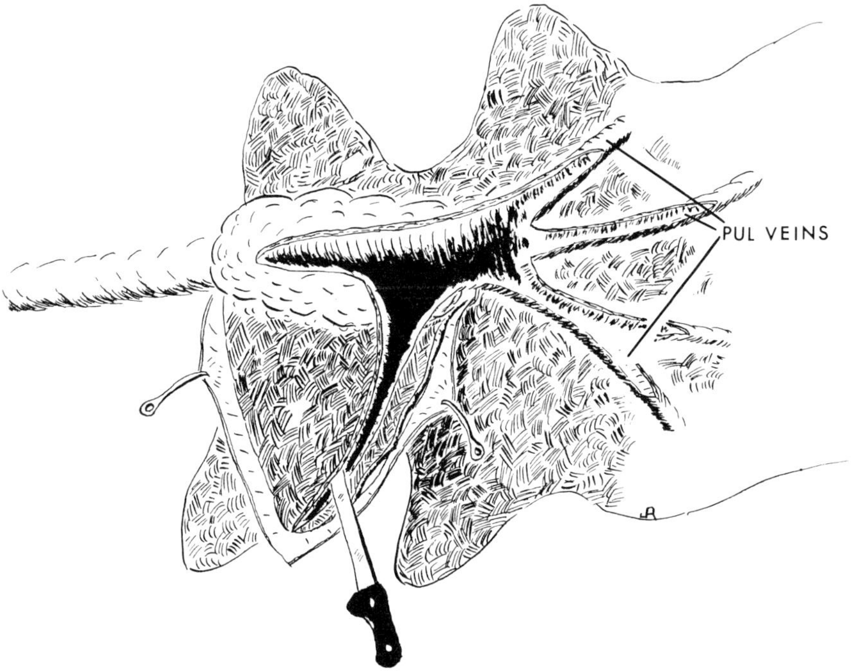

FIG. 81. Pericardium has been reflected. The left atrium has been opened out into the pulmonary veins. The left ventricle is being opened to the apex.

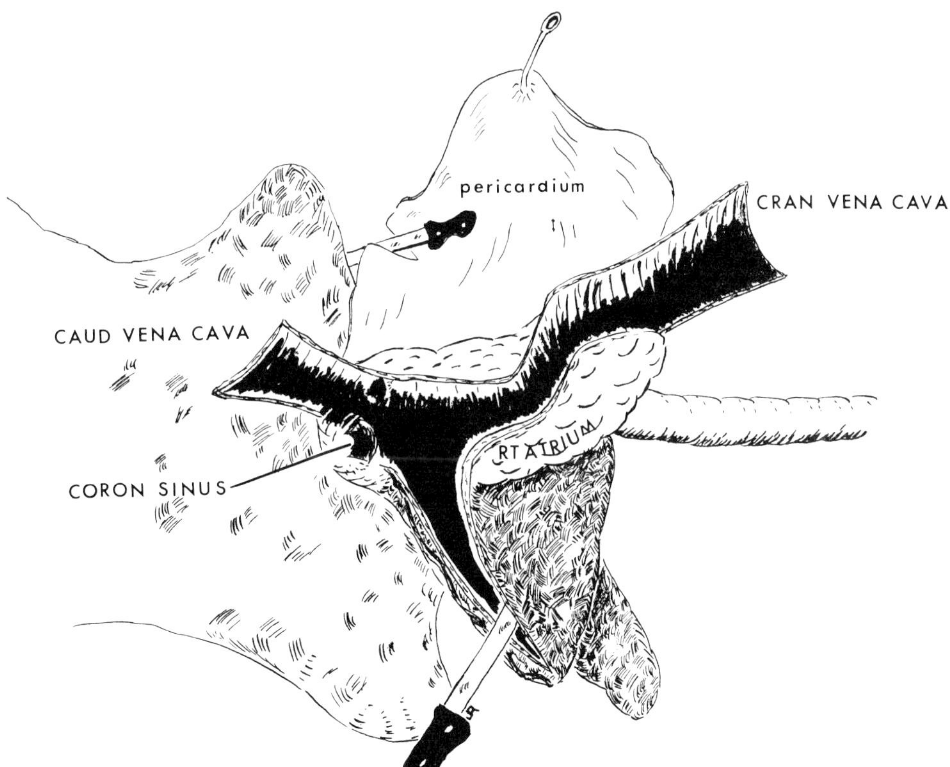

FIG. 82. Heart and lungs reversed. The pericardium is removed. The right atrium, cranial and caudal vena cavae and coronary sinus are opened. The right ventricle is opened (knife) along the right longitudinal groove to the apex. The next cut (*arrow*) will be from the apex, parallel to the left longitudinal groove toward the pulmonary artery.

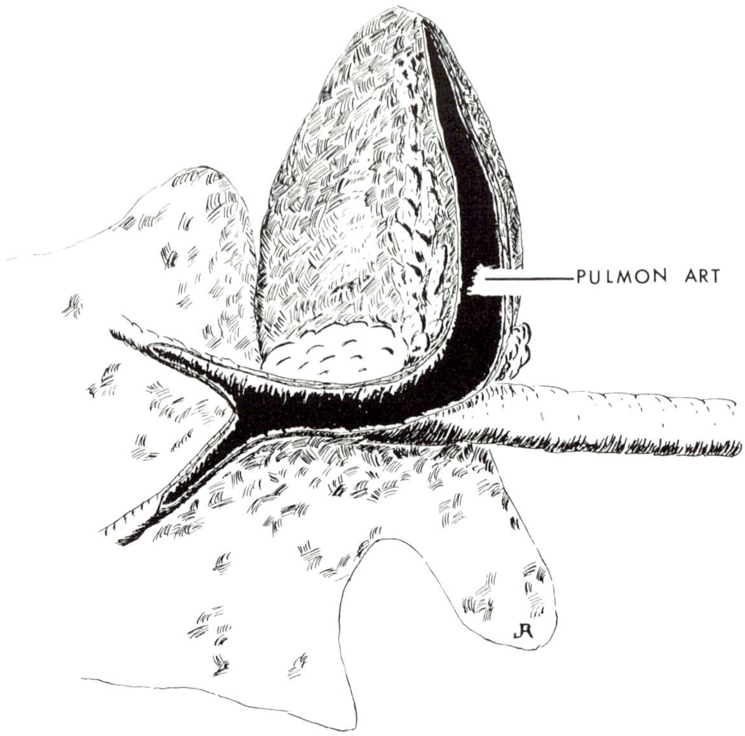

FIG. 83. The apex of the heart is tipped directly away from the prosector and the cut parallel to the left longitudinal groove carried out the pulmonary artery.

monary artery and out the major branches to the right and left lungs (Fig. 83). Note that the pulmonary veins are destroyed as the artery is opened. The heart is now separated from the lungs since all the venous and arterial connections between them have been examined. Grasp both aorta and heart and cut free from the lungs.

With the left ventricle presenting, palpate the aortic orifice by running the finger up under the A-V valve. Introduce the knife in the same manner and cut through the A-V valve and aortic ring, opening the thoracic aorta completely. The ductus arteriosus (or ligamentum arteriosum) should be examined.

Examine the cusps of the aortic valve. Open the right coronary artery from its origin just above the aortic valve, through the coronary groove and down the right longitudinal groove. Open the left coronary artery from its aortic origin, following the descending branch down the left longitudinal groove and the circumflex branch through the coronary groove on the left. When the lumina of the vessels becomes too small for convenient slitting with the knife, one may continue by making serial transverse cuts 2 to 3 mm. apart across the vessels.

Sever all the chordae tendinae, palpate the A-V valve leaflets and make multiple slices into the ventricular musculature.

Interpretation

Pharynx

The lymphoid nodules of the pharynx are prominent in the young animal (29). With acute upper respiratory infection (for example, rhinopneumonitis) the lymphoid tissue may appear more prominent and be ringed by petechial hemorrhages, diffusing into hyperemia of the entire mucosa.

Chronic cough and the causes thereof have not been defined pathologically. The prominent lymphoid nodules frequently described on endoscopic examination as evidence of chronic pharyngitis are probably normal. Although I have never autopsied a horse with known chronic cough, I have never, in a large experience, seen a case of chronic pharyngitis. The acute pharyngitis often associated with viral upper respiratory infections does not seem to become chronic, but rather seems to resolve completely. There is clinical evidence that chronic cough may be a tracheitis or bronchitis. More work remains to be done.

Small, focal abscesses are commonly found in the tonsillar tissues. As a rule these are single or widely separated and consist of pieces of foreign material (straw, hay) imbedded in a tonsillar crypt and surrounded by pus. They are of little or no clinical significance. Occasionally a strangles abscess may involve the tonsillar tissues.

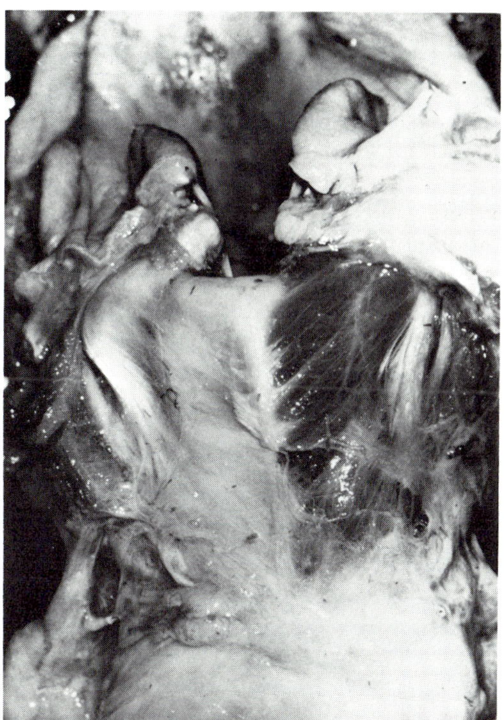

FIG. 84. Dorsal view of the larynx with left cricoarytenoideus dorsalis muscle atrophy.

Esophagus

Esophageal lesions are not common. Fine, often barely perceptible, erosions in the distal third are characteristic of a specific acute-chronic diarrhea in horses (p. 80). More extensive erosions may be seen as a result of stomach tube administration of caustic substances. Frequently, in acute gastric dilatation, there will be massive ulceration of the distal third of the esophagus, presumably as a result of regurgitation of acidic gastric contents. Typically, there is yellowish or yellowish-green discoloration of the erosions and intervening normal mucosa. Warble (*Hypoderma bovis*) migrations may cause marked, yellow gelatinous edema around the esophagus.

Larynx

The cause of one type of "broken wind" is damage to the recurrent nerve, particularly the left nerve, which supplies all the intrinsic nerves of the larynx with the exception of the cricothyroideus. The muscle atrophy following nerve damage is (from most marked to least marked): cricoarytenoideus dorsalis, arytenoideus transversus, cricoarytenoideus lateralis, ventricularis, vocalis (16) (Fig. 84).

The etiology of laryngeal hemiplegia ("roaring") in horses has long eluded a clear explanation (86). However, the following points may be noted.

1. Roaring is the result of atrophy of the intrinsic laryngeal muscles with consequent "dropping" of the arytenoid cartilage, allowing the vocal fold to obstruct the laryngeal airway.

2. Muscle atrophy occurs primarily on the left side and is secondary to damage to the left recurrent nerve. When roaring occurs on the right, it is considered to be secondary to trauma (needle puncture, for

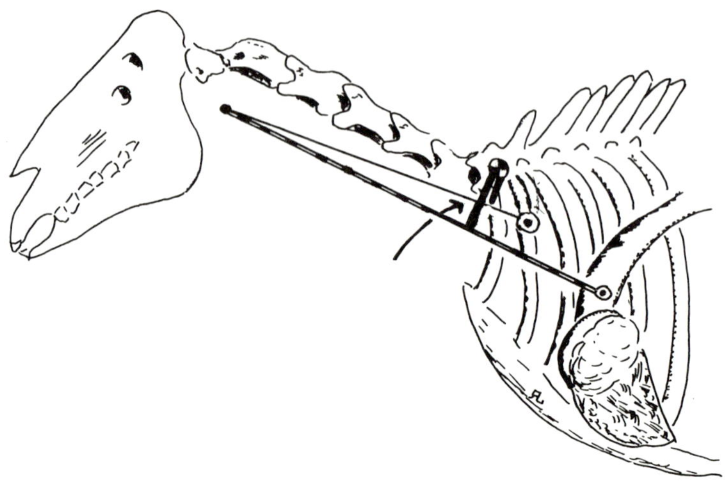

FIG. 85. Left recurrent nerve (*dashed line*) has fixed points at larynx and aortic arch while the right nerve is fixed at the larynx and the costocervical artery. The cervicothoracic junction is indicated by ⊗. The moment arm from the cervicothoracic junction to the left nerve is greater than that to the right nerve. Difference indicated by *arrow*.

example) or some other, definable factor affecting the right recurrent nerve.

3. The primary site of damage to the left recurrent nerve is interpreted to be in the middle third of the nerve (17).

4. Roaring is more common in the larger breeds (draft horses, heavy hunters) and in larger individuals of the light breeds (43).

The left recurrent nerve is longer than the right. It loops around the aortic arch and may be considered fixed at the aortic arch and at the larynx. The right recurrent nerve loops around the costocervical artery and is fixed at this point and at the larynx. The thoracic fixed point of the right recurrent nerve (Fig. 85) is closer to the cervicothoracic junction than the fixed point of the left recurrent nerve. The cervicothoracic junction is the center of rotation (CT) of the head and neck system.

Because of these relationships the left recurrent nerve will be tensed more (tensile force exerted on the nerve) by movement of the head and neck up and/or to the right than the right recurrent nerve when the head and neck are moved up and/or to the left. The left nerve is relaxed when the head and neck move to the left and the right nerve relaxed by movement to the right.

Greater tension will be put on the left nerve of the long neck, large horse than on the left nerve of the shorter neck, small horse, as will be shown below.

These facts are directly related to the relationship between the CT and the thoracic fixed points of the left and right recurrent nerves. The linear force (tension) exerted on the nerve is a function of the torque force exerted on the nerve by movement of the head and neck around the CT. The torque force, in turn, is

$$L = ml^2\alpha$$

where L = torque force, m = mass, l = moment arm, and α = angular acceleration.

The m and α shall be assumed the same for both left and right nerves and large and small horses, leaving only l as a variable.

Although the recurrent nerve is being tensed by movement of the cranial end of the neck (laryngeal fixed point) with the aortic arch or costocervical artery as the thoracic fixed point, the tensile force developed in the nerve is, mechanically, a function of the distance l, where l is the moment arm from the CT to the nerve, l being drawn normal (perpendicular) to the nerve. In Figures 85 and 86, it is obvious that the moment arm of the left recurrent nerve is greater than that of the right recurrent nerve from both the dorsal and lateral aspects.

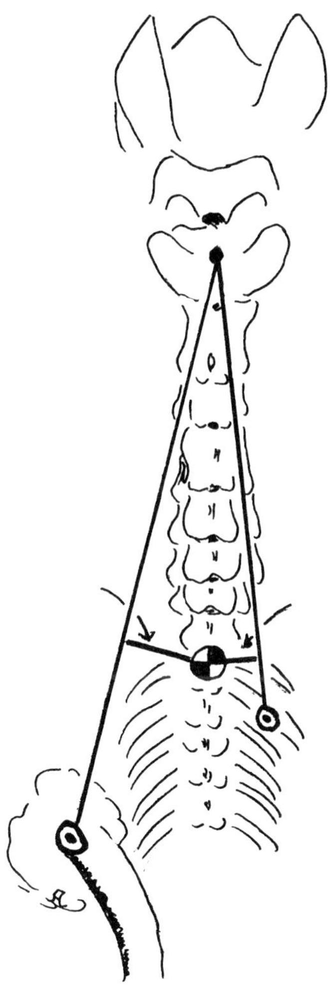

FIG. 86. Dorsal view showing greater moment arm of the left recurrent nerve. *Arrows* point to the moment arms of each nerve.

In Figure 87, the long neck and short neck are compared with the aortic arch remaining stationary relative to the CT. In Figure 88, the relationship of the CT and the aortic arch are changed, with the neck length remaining constant. Figure 87 may be taken to represent a long neck, light horse while Figure 88 represents a moderate, (or even short) neck, large horse. Obviously, the combination of long neck and large horse would provide maximum increase in the moment arm. Figure 89 is the dorsal view of the situation in Figure 87, and Figure 90 is the dorsal view of Figure 88.

The unit tensile force on the left nerve, then, is greater than on the right nerve. Since unit tensile force is

$$S = P/A$$

where S = unit tensile force, P = total tensile force, and A = area of nerve cross section, either P has increased or A has decreased. We have shown that P is larger in the left than the right nerve. When the P force becomes sufficiently large (approaching the limit), however, A, the cross-sectional area, diminishes. That is, the nerve "necks" near the middle, the primary site of damage. This necking would compress blood vessels and compromise the vascular supply in the area of primary damage. This vascular mechanism appears more attractive than direct tensile damage to the nerve fibers.

Thyroid-Parathyroid

The fetus and young foal may show marked enlargement of the thyroid gland with persistence of the thyroglossal duct. (Fig. 91) Histologically, the acini are enlarged and the epithelium flattened. In

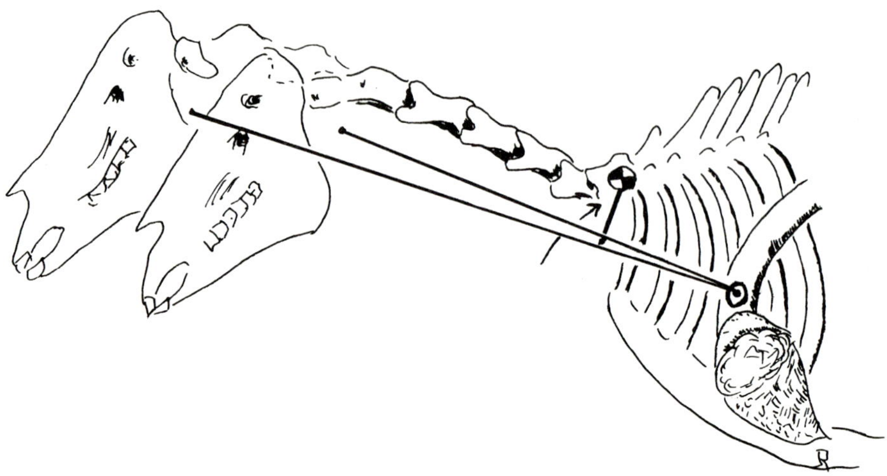

FIG. 87. Long neck and short neck horses compared. The moment arm (*arrow*) of the left recurrent nerve of the long neck horse is greater than that of the short neck horse.

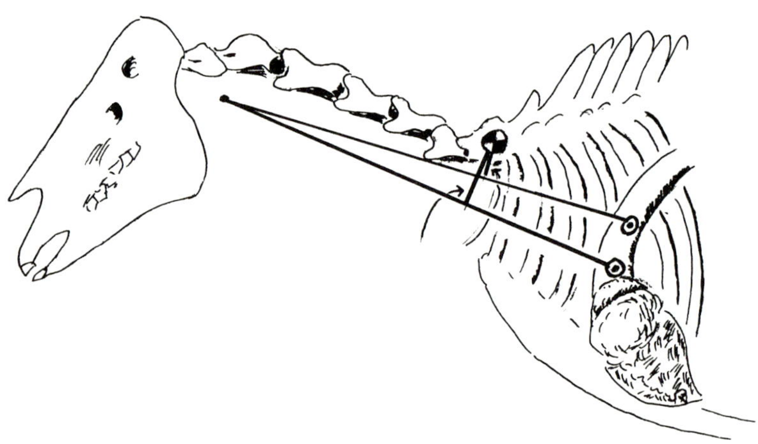

FIG. 88. Increase in moment arm (*arrow*) of deep-bodied horse; aortic arch fixed point is located more ventrally.

most foals the thyroid regresses to normal size by a few months of age without untoward effects. In some cases, however, delayed ossification and crushing of carpal and tarsal bones has been associated with such goiters (59). Recently, evidence has been brought forward that these "congenital" goiters are the result of excessive iodine intake by the mare (4).

Older animals show marked microscopic pigmentation of the acinar epithelium and *dysharmonie*—marked variation in acinar size. Hyperplastic or adenomatous nodules, white or tan and of widely varying size, progressively increase in frequency, size, and number with advancing age. The endocrine effects, if any, of these changes are not known.

Both internal (IV) and external (III) parathyroid glands are present. They are coarsely or finely lobulated and may contain cysts. Their significance in nutritional secondary hyperparathyroidism has been classically defined (55).

Heart

The significance of the shape of the heart and the relative content of blood in the several chambers of the heart are not easy to resolve and can become quite vexing. From the description which follows it

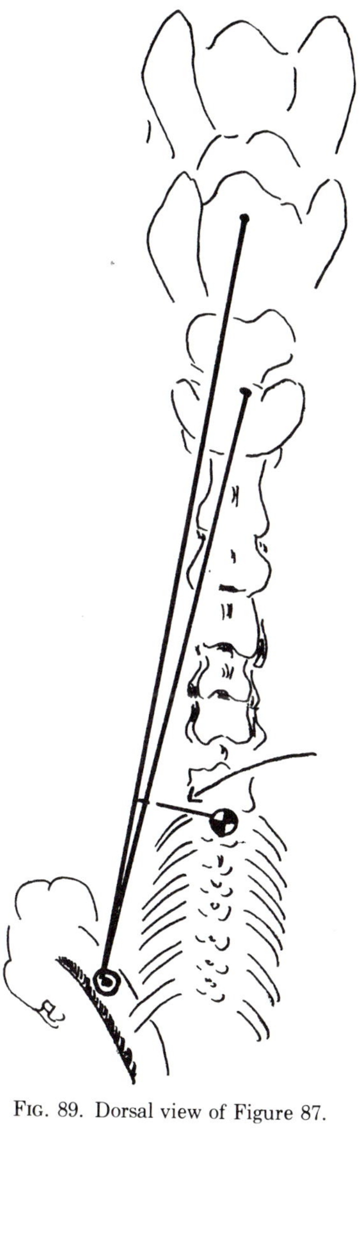

FIG. 89. Dorsal view of Figure 87.

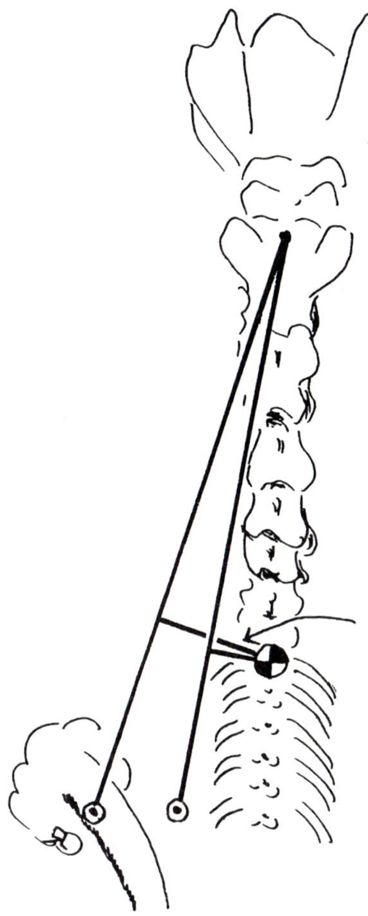

FIG. 90. Dorsal view of Figure 88.

will become apparent that many factors interact to determine the condition of the heart at any given moment after death. All too often one will not be able to determine precisely, or even roughly, what significance, if any, should be attributed to blood in one ventricle or the other or to overall heart shape. It is always best to underinterpret if in doubt. The microscope will make the decision about the presence or absence of myocarditis and the prosector need not be too vexed that he cannot decide whether the flabby left ventricle is antemortem or postmortem.

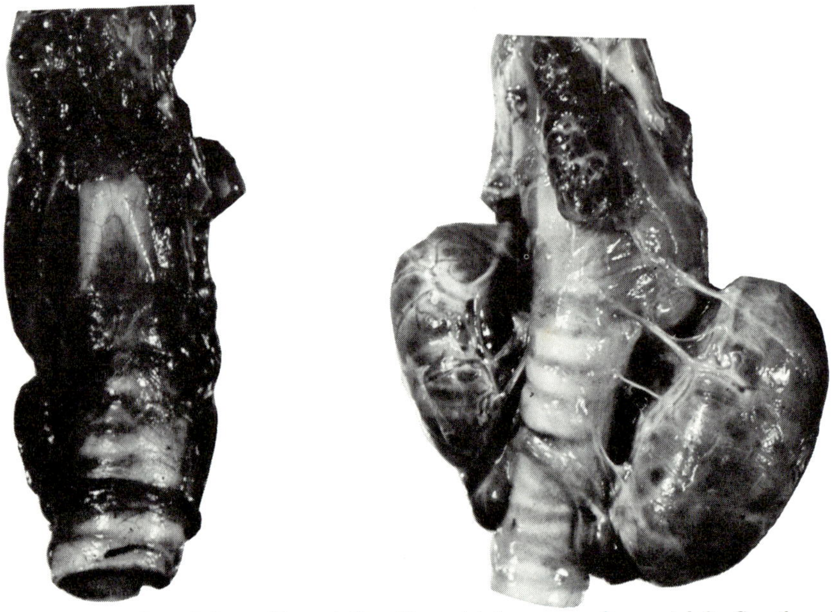

FIG. 91. Goiter in an aborted fetus. Normal thyroids and isthmus are shown at left. Greatly enlarged thyroids and prominent thyroglossal duct with cystic formations are shown at right.

If a normal horse is destroyed, the left ventricle, immediately after death, will be contracted while the right ventricle may or may not be contracted. Within a few minutes both ventricles are strongly in rigor. Soon, and the time will vary considerably, the right ventricle loses rigor and dilates, becoming flabby. Since the right ventricular musculature is thinner than the left, blood is never completely evacuated during rigor, and additional blood may run in from the atrium and pulmonary artery as rigor wanes.

The left ventricle remains tightly contracted until marked decomposition is apparent throughout the carcass. Then, it too dilates, and blood may run in from the atrium and aorta. At this stage it is quite obvious that advanced postmortem changes have occurred, and one cannot determine whether the left ventricular dilatation is postmortem or antemortem.

This basic, "normal" death pattern can be modified greatly by antemortem and agonal events. In the case of virtually any asphyxial, toxic death, the right ventricle will not go into rigor or will go only into weak rigor. The left ventricle will usually go into rigor, but it may not be as marked as usual nor persist as long into the postmortem period. Only in cases of cardiac disease will the left ventricle be frankly dilated at and shortly after death.

Chicken-fat clot, as is well known, indicates a prolonged agonal period with gradual, nonspecific slowing and failure of the heart.

Endocardial and epicardial hemorrhages, whether petechial or ecchymotic, are the rule rather than the exception in any type of death. They indicate only asphyxia and circulatory failure and nothing more. Such hemorrhages acquire significance as indicators of cardiac disease only if they extend a considerable distance into the underlying myocardium. One wearies of journal reports and letters describing endocardial and epicardial hemorrhages in vivacious, useless detail.

Pericardial effusion is uncommon in

horses except in the presence of heart disease and in "shaker foals." I shall digress here to describe so-called shaker foal.

While the clinical signs are variable, most cases can be readily diagnosed on initial examination. There is sudden onset of severe muscular weakness and prostration in a 3- to 8-week-old foal. The foal may be found down and unable to rise several hours after appearing completely normal. When helped to its feet, it may stand for some minutes and nurse. Generalized muscular trembling begins, and the foal drops to the ground as if struck on the head by an axe; the trembling immediately stops. While down the foal may appear normal, follow movements in the stall, and react to pinching.

After lying quietly for some time the animal may rise with assistance, only to tremble and drop again within seconds. As a rule, complete prostration soon develops, and the foal is unable to stand even with assistance. In severe cases trembling may never be observed; the animal is prostrate and unable to stand even with assistance when first observed.

There is complete cessation of peristalsis (ileus), and the pupils are dilated, reacting sluggishly to light. The duration of illness is variable, but with average care death usually occurs within 72 hours.

The most characteristic autopsy changes are: the dorsal and ventral colon are contracted, contain only small quantities of dry, hard ingesta, and have patchy mucosal hyperemia and hemorrhage. There is dry, firm ingesta coated with thick, tenacious mucus in the descending colon. The pericardial sac, in most cases, contains an excessive amount of clear, yellow fluid with variable quantities of free fibrin flakes and strands. There is diffuse petechiation of the epicardium. For further details, etiological considerations, etc., see the original publication (76).

I have only seen one case of fibrinous pericarditis in a foal, caused by *Corynebacterium pyogenes*.

The atria are remarkably free of lesions. Small lipomas may be found hanging from the epicardial fat in animals of all ages. In older horses there is occasionally an irregular, focal, transmural scarring of the right atrium. I have not seen the bone formation which has been described (69). Microscopically, the lesion is composed of fibrous tissue and chronic inflammatory cell infiltration. The cause is unknown, and I do not know whether atrial arrythmias and/or electrocardiographic changes accompany the developing or developed lesion. This lesion may be confused with nontransmural focal epicardial fibrosis and/or fatty infiltration.

Congenital cardiac anomalies are not common in horses but do occur. Table 1 summarizes the reported cases. It may be noted that a double origin of the left coronary artery from the aorta is not uncommon and is of no pathological significance. Blood- or serum-filled cysts may be present in the A-V valves of foals, although much less frequently than in calves. They represent persistent segments of the fetal valvular blood vessels (16).

In the young foal the foramen ovale is covered by a cylindrical, fishnet-like structure (finger of a lady's lace glove) which can be pushed into the left atrium on the little finger. As a general rule the foramen is anatomically sealed about one month of age.

The ductus arteriosus remains probe-patent for a variable period of time after birth but, in general, is anatomically closed by the second month. The position of the ligamentum arteriosum is marked by irregular depressed areas on the intimal surfaces of both the aorta and pulmonary artery.

Fenestration of the aortic valve margins is regularly seen. I do not believe that it is completely clear (62) whether the holes

TABLE 1
Cardiac Anomalies in Horses

No. of Cases	Diagnosis	Author*
2†	Pericardial defect	Forgeot; Gaddi
1	Cor triloculare biatriatum, stenosis of conus pulmonalis	Awtokratow
1	Persistent truncus arteriosus; subaortic septal defect, atresia right A-V ostium, truncus from right ventricle	Brandt
1	Persistent truncus arteriosus; truncus over-riding subaortic septal defect	Lilleengen
1	Persistent truncus arteriosus; subaortic septal defect, truncus from right ventricle	Lilleengen
1	Ostium atrioventricular communis	Berg
9	Subaortic septal defects	Biernacki; Preisz; Czokor; Lupke; Walley; Lilleengen
1	Rokitansky defect	Aellig
2	Intertrabecular septal defect	Walley; Hutyra
1†	Aortic stenosis, subaortic septal defect, intertrabecular septal defect, patent ductus arteriosus, 2 valve leaflets—aortic and right A-V	Hutyra
1	Double vena cava	Leisering
1	6 leaflet left A-V valve	Goedecke
1	Left A-V leaflet enlarged 3× and perforated	Behrens
1	A-V ostium (not specified), a central perforated membrane	Kitt
6	Malformation—aortic, pulmonary valves; pulmonary—2 leaflets Aortic—2 leaflets Aortic—5 leaflets	Cadiot; Lazitchs; Mollman Hutyra† Czokor
2	Right A-V atresia, subaortic septal defect, patent foramen ovale	Rooney and Frank
1	Absence of aortic origin left coronary artery	Rooney and Frank
1	Persistent truncus arteriosus	Rooney and Frank
1	Persistent ductus arteriosus	Rooney and Frank

* See Rooney and Frank (87).
† Donkey.

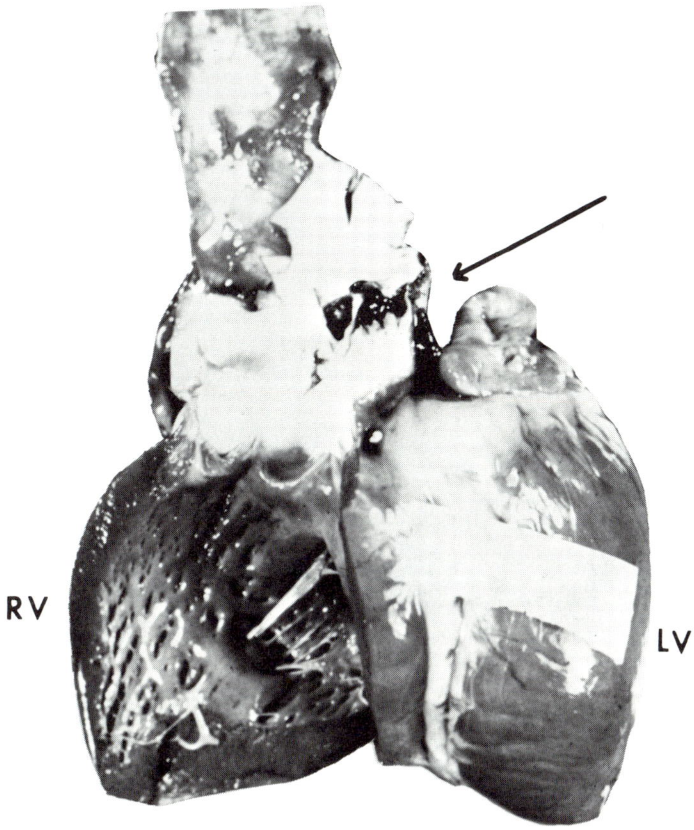

FIG. 92. Rupture of pulmonary artery in a foal. The photo was somewhat overexposed to emphasize the tear.

are present antemortem. In any event this "lesion" is not associated with clinical signs, and is of no pathological significance.

Rupture of the pulmonary artery has been seen once in an adult horse and on several occasions in young foals. The rupture so completely disrupts the wall of the artery that one cannot be certain (Fig. 92) that a congenital mural defect was present in any given case, but that is presumed.

Often, in young foals, there is mural calcification in the pulmonary artery (as well as in aorta, carotids and limb arteries), which is further evidence for mural defects predisposing to rupture.

Rupture of the aorta is of two types (79). In the classical type the rupture occurs above the level of the aortic valves and death quickly results from cardiac tamponade. In the second type, confined to breeding stallions, the rupture occurs near or at the aortic ring below the origin of the right coronary artery (Figs. 93 and 94). Death may be rapid because, presumably, of interruption of the A-V bundle. In many cases the blood dissects through to the right ventricle, forming a cardioaortic fistula; death follows a variably prolonged period of clinically obvious cardiac failure. The clinical history is characteristic: sud-

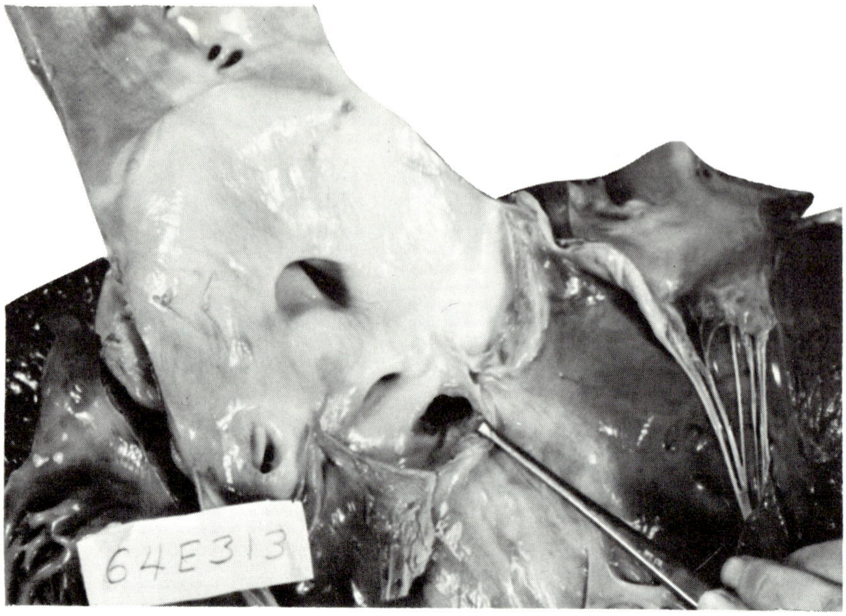

FIG. 93. Aortic ring rupture just below the right coronary orifice. (Photograph reused courtesy of *Pathologica Veterinaria*.)

den death or heart failure signs after breeding, especially early in the breeding season. Clinical examination of the heart reveals severe tachycardia and, in some cases at least, a murmur may be detected in the area of the aortic valve. At autopsy the tear may be quite small and can be easily overlooked unless the area behind the aortic valve cusp is specifically examined.

Vegetative endocarditis (103) occurs occasionally, involving the left A-V valve and/or the aortic valve. The clinical course is often protracted with variable ventral edema and fluctuating temperature. Streptococci have always been the cause in my experience. Embolization may occur. I have only seen endocarditis of the right A-V valve on one occasion, related to cardioaortic fistula.

With age there is an increased incidence of thickening and scarring of the aortic valves. This must not be confused with the small fibrous nodules normally present at the center of the free border of each valve cusp. Such scarring may be associated with clinical signs, although very often it is an incidental finding at autopsy. The cause is unknown but in some cases, at least, the scarring may be ascribed to prior, healed endocarditis; in most cases, however, it appears to be simply a phenomenon of aging.

The free edges of the A-V valves, similarly, tend to become thicker and more irregular with age. It seems clear enough that this is wear and tear not related to prior endocarditis (at least for the right A-V valve).

Myocardial lesions do occur. In older animals focal areas of fibrosis, one to numerous, may be found in the myocardium. Microscopic study provides no real clue to their cause, but presumably they are the healed remnants of an earlier focal myocarditis.

Acute focal or diffuse myocarditis may

be seen as isolated lesions or in association with upper respiratory infection, notably strangles and influenza. There are degenerative changes in the muscle fibers (myolysis) and focal, interstitial edema, and round cell infiltration. A few cases of pure streptococcal myocarditis have been seen (at least presumed pure on the basis of culture and finding of the organisms in sections together with a neutrophile infiltrate). Most isolated cases would appear to be of viral origin but, to date, virological studies have been only sketchily and inadequately performed.

In man there is considerable evidence that myocardial changes may accompany a variety of pathological processes in other regions of the body. Such correlations have not been clearly defined pathologically in horses and more routine histological examination of the heart is definitely required.

Coronary disease and occlusion are vir-

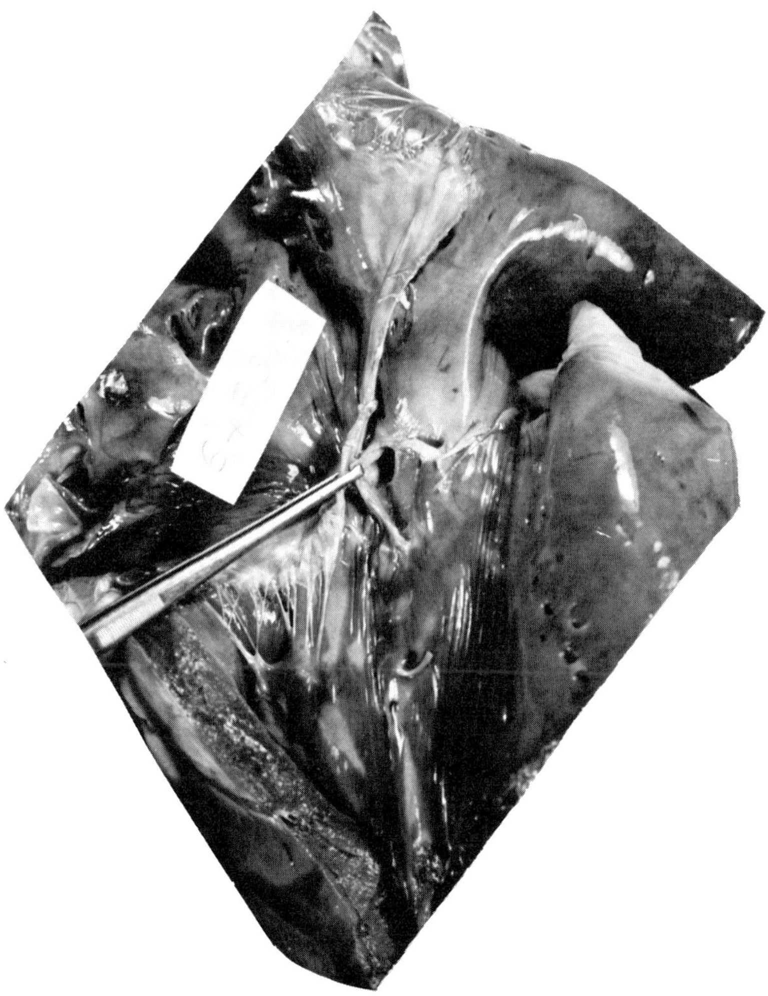

FIG. 94. Opening into the right ventricle of a cardioaortic fistula as a result of aortic ring rupture. (Photograph reused courtesy of *Pathologica Veterinaria*.)

tually unknown in the horse. Very rarely, aberrant *S. vulgaris* larvae may cause thrombosis near the root of the aorta with embolization into the coronaries.

Two unsettling conditions remain for consideration. Partial and complete heart-block have been well described clinically and electrically. The morphological bases, if any, are unknown. Exquisitely detailed autopsy studies of such cases are urgently needed.

The second condition is nameless but may be called idiopathic cardiac dilatation. I have autopsied several animals with an obvious clinical history of heart failure. At autopsy, immediately after death, there was symmetrical cardiac dilatation. Microscopically, there were lesions of "myocardosis" (96)—early, minimal myofiber necrosis, interstitial edema and hyperemia. The cause was not determined in any of these cases.

For further discussion of cardiac problems, see Detweiler and Patterson (20).

TEN

The Lungs

Dissection

Orient the lungs on the table with the dorsal surfaces uppermost. Slice and examine the left and right bronchial lymph nodes and the caudal mediastinal lymph nodes. Carefully examine the pleural surfaces of the lungs. Open the trachea and the major bronchi. Make multiple transverse slices through the lung and carefully examine and palpate all the slices.

Interpretation

Small focal lesions in the lungs not apparent to the naked eye can be detected by palpation. In the presence of advanced postmortem changes true consolidation is readily differentiated by palpation. There may be black or blackish-green anthracotic discoloration of the bronchial lymph nodes in older animals as well as atrophy of the lymphoid tissue.

As a rule the lungs collapse quickly when the diaphragm is opened. The surface will be somewhat wrinkled. The normally thicker, whitish pleura over the dorsal part of the diaphragmatic portions of the lungs will appear even thicker because of the collapse. If the lungs do not collapse, the reason should be ascertained immediately. Often, although not invariably, the lungs will be distended with air and not collapse for a considerable period of time when an animal has been euthanized. The lungs of an animal afflicted with "heaves" will not collapse but will, in fact, be greatly distended by alveolar emphysema and bear rib impressions. Lungs affected by edema and pneumonia do not collapse normally. Postmortem as well as antemortem edema will prevent collapse.

Agonal changes are common and must be differentiated from lesions significantly involved in the clinical disease. Bright petechiae and patchy hemorrhages on the pleural surface and deep in the parenchyma are usually agonal. There may be uneven, patchy emphysema, with bullous distension near the margins and patchy, raised whitish plaques elsewhere.

If the animal was in lateral recumbency or dorsal recumbency (surgical procedures) for some time before death, there will be hypermia and extravasation of blood in the dependent portions of the lungs. Such hypostatic congestion also occurs after death.

Pulmonary edema as an antemortem, nonagonal event is uncommon in horses. Postmortem edema, on the other hand, is common. The two are differentiated by the presence of foam in the bronchi and trachea in the case of antemortem and agonal edema and the absence of foam with postmortem edema.

Antemortem edema as a nonagonal clinical event occurs (1) together with pneumonia, (2) as a result of massive fluid therapy, and (3) following severe brain trauma. In the case of fluid therapy it is hardly possible to cause pulmonary edema by oral or intravenous administration in normal animals. The excess fluid is cleared by renal action almost as fast as it is administered. On one occasion a researcher tried to produce water intoxication in a horse. Simple deprivation followed by free access to water produced no clinical signs. He then pumped water in by stomach tube. While he perspired and pumped away, the horse ran water from the penis in an almost steady stream. Sweat puddled around the man and urine beneath the horse. The experiment was abandoned.

In a sick animal intravenous fluids can cause pulmonary edema. It would appear that damage to the pulmonary capillaries as a result of acidosis may play a significant role. If severe acidosis of the pulmonary vascular bed is produced experimentally by jugular infusion of acetic acid, severe pulmonary edema quickly develops.

The mechanism of pulmonary edema following brain trauma is not known. Severe traumatic damage to the brain (fracture and/or hemorrhage) of horses will often be followed by pulmonary edema if the animal survives for some hours.

Atelectasis as a significant clinical and pathological process is uncommon except in young foals. Areas of atelectasis occur in relation to bronchiolitis and pneumonia as well as, on a larger scale, with massive pleuritis. The process is quite overshadowed, however, by the primary lesions.

It is difficult to enter upon a meaningful discussion of the gross pathology of the several varieties of equine pneumonia. Let it be clearly understood, therefore, that what follows is in the nature of generalization.

Inhalation pneumonia is not uncommon, particularly in foals fed by stomach tube. The usual cause is overloading of the stomach with regurgitation into the respiratory tract. If the case is uncomplicated by bacterial infection, there will be focal areas of plum-red consolidation, particularly in the right lung, which can easily be mistaken for atelectasis. Rarely, there may be inadvertent infusion of, or regurgitation of, oil into the lungs causing a chronic, focal, fibrosing pneumonia. The bronchial lymph nodes may contain lipid-laden macrophages.

Meconium aspiration is apparently a normal phenomenon; at least it is a very common phenomenon in the newborn foal (83). As a rule, meconium elicits very little or no inflammatory reaction. If a bacterial agent, particularly streptococcus, invades the lung, however, a severe fibrinous pneumonia develops which may mistakenly be attributed to meconium alone.

Three distinct types of viral pneumonia have been recognized, to date, in the horse. Fetal rhinopneumonitis is discussed in detail in Chapter 11. A number of foals are born alive, at term, with intrauterine rhinopneumonitis infection. They are in severe respiratory distress at birth, do not respond to therapy, and usually die within 24 to 48 hours. The gross appearance of the lungs is startling and characteristic. There are wide bands of interlobular yellow, gelatinous edema outlining a mosaic patch-work of consolidated, plum-red lobules and white, bulging emphysematous lobules. As a rule, in contrast to the aborted fetus, pleural effusion is minimal.

Recently an adenovirus has been found which causes pneumonia in foals one month or older (all cases to date have been in Arabians). The gross lung specimen has focal to confluent plum-red consolidation. Microscopically, the lesions closely resemble those of rhinopneumonitis. The age difference is, however, characteristic.

I have not seen influenzal pneumonia at autopsy in older horses. Several fatal cases were seen in foals, however, when the A2 strain of virus first reached the breeding farms. In the few cases uncomplicated by secondary bacterial invasion the lungs had plum-red consolidation with excess, thick, mucoid material in the smaller bronchi. The microscopic picture was characteristic of that seen in influenza in many species.

Bacterial pneumonias are not uncommon, particularly in foals. Shigella and streptococcal septicemias are usually accompanied by pneumonia. In more acute cases the pneumonic process is hemorrhagic in nature, whereas with more prolonged cases of streptococcal infection abscessation becomes a prominent feature.

Fibrinous pneumonia is rare with the exception of contagious pleuropneumonia; most cases of pneumonia in horses are bronchopneumonia. The gross appearance of the lung will vary from intense hyperemia with barely palpable consolidation to scattered focal areas of consolidation to focal, confluent consolidation. Purulent material is almost always expressible from the bronchi and bronchioles.

The interacting role of viruses and bacteria in causing pneumonia is unclear. Although the gross, microscopic, and bacteriological studies may clearly point to a pure bacterial process, one is always concerned that a virus may have initiated the pathological process. Microscopic examination of the lungs may not reveal subtle viral changes overshadowed by the purulent, necrotizing bacterial process. It is always useful to examine the nasal mucosa, in particular the nasal septum, microscopically. There may be erosive lesions and rhinitis suggestive of viral infection, and these lesions will usually not be masked by secondary bacterial infection.

C. equi (61) causes either an enzootic or sporadic disease problem in foals. The clinical disease may take several forms which are clearly mirrored in the pathological findings.

Peracute pneumonia is an uncommon form; the apparently normal foal is found dead or dies very shortly after the onset of severe respiratory difficulty. At autopsy both lungs are extensively consolidated, firm, dark plum-red with only minimal mucoid to mucopurulent bronchial exudate. Histological study shows an acute, diffuse purulent pneumonia. This form is apparently the result of massive, overwhelming exposure.

Acute pneumonia with dyspnea and elevated temperature is more common. Standard antibiotic therapy does not remarkably change the clinical course during the first 48 to 72 hours after onset, and the disease is either fatal or assumes a more chronic form. If death occurs at this stage, there will usually be a diffuse pneumonia characterized by multiple pinhead to pea-sized or larger abscesses with a cheesy, caseous content.

Chronic pneumonia is the most common form of the disease in my experience. After an acute onset, which may be so slight as to pass almost unnoticed, the animal gradually loses weight and condition and has variably severe respiratory signs. If the infection involves the large intestine, as it does in a small number of cases, diarrhea may be a feature. The animal gradually declines, and at autopsy there will be multiple large abscesses scattered throughout the lungs (Fig. 95) and perhaps also in the colic lymph nodes and colon mucosa. Often the chronically ill animal dies suddenly and unexpectedly. At autopsy large abscesses are present as well as diffuse consolidation of the type

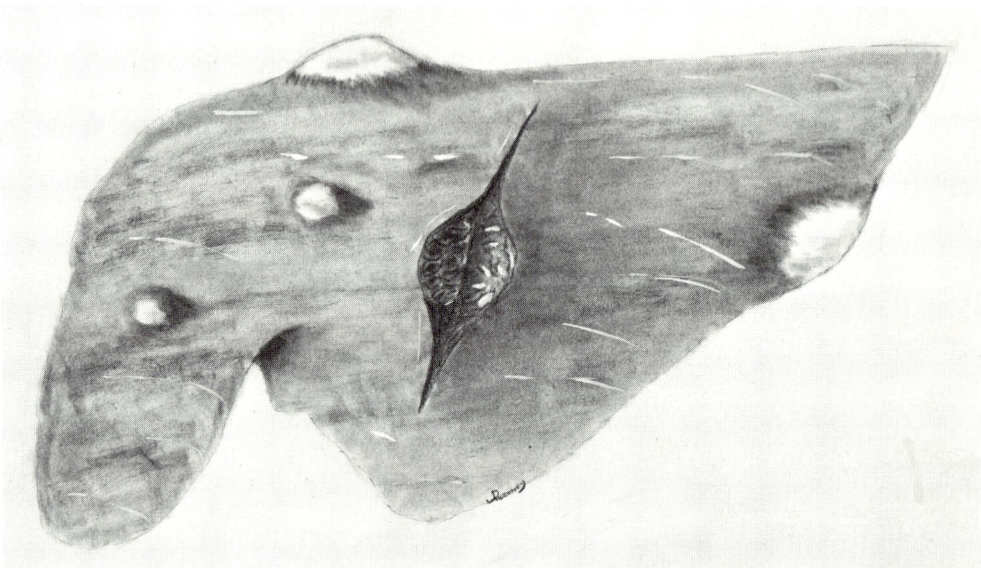

FIG. 95. Multiple abscesses in lung, one sliced open.

seen in the peracute disease. This may be sudden miliary dissemination from one or more of the large abscesses.

One may, rarely, find a single *C. equi* abscess in the lung of an older, debilitated animal. Age apparently confers strong resistance against *C. equi*. It appears to be a poorly invasive pathogen which selects weak or debilitated individuals. While outbreaks in large groups of young animals have been reported from Sweden and Australia epizootics occur only among Arabian foals in the United States.

Pleuritis is a common, debilitating, and fatal disease. It is primarily a disease of the traveling horse. An acute upper respiratory disease appears to resolve, and the horse is either put back in training or shipped while still convalescing. A secondary streptococcal upper respiratory disease appears with a copious purulent nasal discharge, fever, and debilitation. Recovery from this second episode may appear uneventful, and the horse may again be either shipped or trained. Pleuritis develops. The secondary bacterial upper respiratory infection may be so slight or overlap so that it is not observed or not distinguished from the primary, viral disease. Pleuritis, of course, can occur in any event.

In virtually all cases of pleuritis there is, in addition to (Fig. 26) the massive serofibrinopurulent effusion in the chest cavity, a focal streptococcal abscess in the lung. This abscess, arising during the secondary upper respiratory infection described above, provides the nidus for the pleural infection. It may be large and readily located or quite small and detectable only by careful palpation of the entire lung, particularly the middle lobe of the right lung. Typically, the abscess has a grayish, watery, flocculent content.

While somewhat out of place, the nature of abscess contents in general requires mention. With experience a reasonable guess as to the nature of the responsible organism can be made on the basis of the location of the abscess and its content. *S.*

equi, usually located in the neck, has a creamy, yellow content. *C. equi*, usually in the lung and large intestine, generally induces a cheesy, whitish, caseous exudate. The common streptococcus abscess may vary considerably in both location and content, in part because there are undoubtedly a number of different pathogenic strains. On average, however, the content tends to be watery, grayish, and flocculent.

Two bizarre cases of pleuritis may be noted. In one a pea-sized stone had been inhaled, causing a focal area of bronchiectasis and abscessation followed by pleuritis. In the second case a 30-cm. multiflora rose branch had been inhaled, perforated the right diaphragmatic part of the lung and the adjacent diaphragm and initiated pleuritis.

"Tracks" of subpleural hemorrhage may occasionally be encountered, particularly on the dorsal part of the lung. They are caused by migration of the ox warble (*H. bovis*), although the warble may have moved on by the time of autopsy.

Firm nodules of variable size are common beneath the pleura and deep in the lungs. Discrete, round grayish nodules in young horses are usually normal lymphoid nodules which regress with age. Hard, fibrous nodules in horses of any age are histologically composed of fibrous tissue, round cells, and variable numbers of eosinophiles. Occasionally, *Aspergillus* sp. hyphae may be present. It appears that these lesions are the result of parasite larval migrations which may be secondarily infected by *Aspergillus*. It should be noted that *Aspergillus* can almost always be cultured from the respiratory tract of the horse and can set up secondary infection whenever the opportunity presents.

Larger and/or more irregularly demarcated masses generally are areas of focal, chronic, interstitial, proliferative pneumonia (so-called adenomatosis) (83). Usually the lesions are of such chronicity that no cause can be determined (except in the case of focal lipid pneumonia). Neither of these lesions, parasitic nodules or chronic, focal pneumonia, are of known clinical significance.

"Heaves," chronic pulmonary emphysema, is readily recognized clinically and at autopsy. The lungs will not collapse, as they contain large quantities of air, and they will appear whiter than normal. The basic lesion (acute, then chronic bronchiolitis causing partial or complete obstruction of the more distal airways) is not usually appreciable grossly. Although arguments persist in some quarters, it seems clear that the emphysema is secondary to bronchiolar obstruction in turn caused by an allergic bronchiolitis (42, 99).

Bleeding in racehorses (epistaxis) is a common and vexing problem. Several causes have been suggested: (1) guttural pouch mycosis; (2) acute hemorrhagic pneumonia; (3) bleeding "points" in the mucosae of the upper respiratory passages; and (4) pulmonary hemorrhage without pneumonia.

Guttural pouch mycosis has been discussed and is well established as a cause of epistaxis (Fig. 50). I have seen several cases of acute hemorrhagic pneumonia, associated with shipping and apparently caused by streptococci (although a primary virus etiology was not eliminated). These several cases had epistaxis before death. In a few instances apparently normal horses were worked or raced. Soon after work, epistaxis occurred and was followed by a fatal, fulminant, hemorrhagic pneumonia.

Bleeding points in the mucosae may or may not occur. There is no autopsy evidence to support such a cause. The ap-

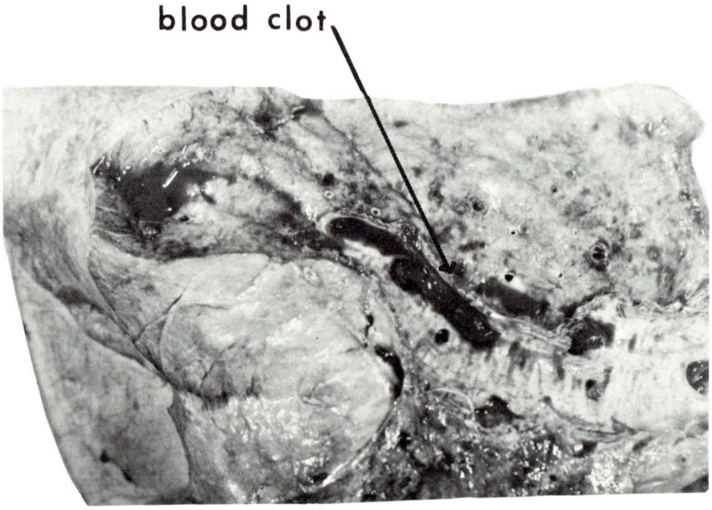

FIG. 96. Clot of blood in bronchus in the diaphragmatic lobe of the lung of a horse which went through a protracted agonal period.

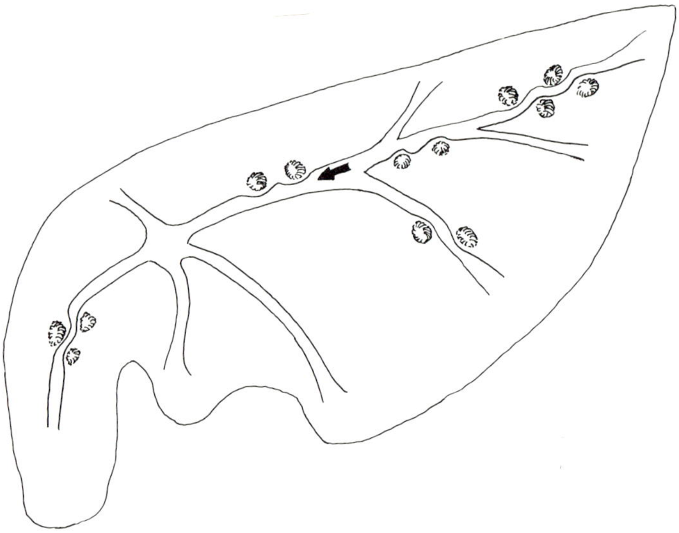

FIG. 97. Diagram to indicate the obstruction of the venous return from the lung by distended air spaces. The greatest distance, and therefore the greatest total obstruction, would be of the venous return from the dorsal part of the diaphragmatic lobe.

pearance of flecks of blood through the laryngoscope does not constitute sufficient evidence.

Pulmonary hemorrhage may well be the most important and common cause of epistaxis. The evidence may be summarized:

1. During the agonal period, asphyxial hemorrhages are common in the lungs. If the agonal period is prolonged, streams of blood will be found in the bronchi and even the trachea and larynx. It is clear that free blood can stream up the airway

without admixing significantly with the air stream (Fig. 96). The assumption that pulmonary hemorrhage will always appear as blood-tinged foam is not true.

2. Sparks (95) has shown that horses, particularly when breaking rapidly from the starting gate, may hold their breath for 30 seconds or more. When such animals finally take a breath, they may either stop or bleed, or both.

3. One autopsy has been performed on a horse with a history of recurrent epistaxis with the last episode within a month of autopsy (36). There was a marked greenish discoloration of the dorsocaudal portions of the diaphragmatic lobes of both lungs. Histologically, these areas were characterized by numerous hemosiderophages and elastotic degenerative changes of pulmonary veins.

The evidence may be interpreted as follows:

Epistaxis results from pulmonary hemorrhage which is caused by asphyxiation in turn caused by breath-holding. The diaphragmatic lobe localization may be rationalized as follows. The horse takes a deep breath and holds it, distending the air spaces. The distended air spaces (distended for a longer period than normal) compromise the flow of blood through the thin-walled pulmonary veins. As shown in Figure 97 the stasis of blood should be most marked at the greatest distance from the point of exit of the venous blood from the lung parenchyma and, therefore, the histological changes in the pulmonary veins (evidence of overdistension) should be in the dorsocaudal portion of the diaphragamatic lobes.

In several cases of massive epistaxis and death following a workout or race, the pulmonary hemorrhage involved large areas of the lung and not the diaphragmatic lobes alone. This is quite reasonable. Moderate asphyxia will involve the diaphragmatic lobes (the most sensitive anatomicofunctional area) while more severe degrees of asphyxia will progressively involve more and more lung area.

The basic cause of most cases of racehorse epistaxis, then, may be asphyxia, whether caused by breath-holding alone or by other causes such as partial obstruction of the airway by laryngeal hemiplegia, tumors, or whatever.

ELEVEN

The Fetus and Foal

Examination of the aborted fetus, fetal membranes, and the term foal presents a somewhat different set of problems than that of the postnatal animal. Since there appears to be no recent compilation of these problems in the equine, they are discussed at length in this chapter. At the outset, the reader must accept that there will be much generalization. It is an unpleasant fact of life that many fetuses die and decompose in the uterus before being expelled, and there is very little one can do, as a pathologist, to ascertain the cause of death and abortion. This short treatise is not meant to be the only or last word. It represents seven years of experience with abortions and aborted fetuses, codifies what is known or seems known, and clearly exposes to view the wide, fascinating vistas of abyssmal ignorance.

Dissection

The exenteration and examination procedure used for fetuses and term foals should be similar to that for postnatal animal. All too often, the fetus is frankly decomposed and the usual exenteration procedure is not worth the effort which must be expended. In such cases the fetus is placed in dorsal recumbency, and all four legs laid down. Starting at the manubrium sterni, the entire ventral surface of the body is removed with the knife. The cervical and throat regions are dissected, as has been described. The thoracic and abdominal viscera are examined *in situ*.

Interpretation

For didactic purposes the embryonic-fetal losses are divided into four overlapping periods. No scientific brief is made for this division; it is solely a framework for the discussion. The periods are: (1) early abortion; (2) four- to six-month abortion; (3) six- to eleven-month abortion; and (4) term foal.

Early Abortion

Abortions, from conception to about the fourth month of gestation, are rarely observed, leading to the erroneous idea that fetal resorption has occurred. I do not believe that such resorption ever occurs. Occasionally a fetus will be expelled only as far as the vagina and decompose before being expelled in an unrecognizable or unrecognized form. Mummification has not been observed except in twins. The failure to observe early abortions is largely due to the small size of the conceptus, husbandry conditions, and the relative ease and rapidity with which the mare aborts.

Approximately 5 to 8% of mares in foal at 45 days will be barren (have aborted) at 150 days (91). Despite the significance of such an abortion rate very little is known of the cause or causes. I have had an opportunity to examine only seven fetuses aborted during this period. All were partially decomposed, yielded pure cultures of streptococci or a mixed bacterial flora, and histologically showed saturation of all tissues with bacteria without an inflammatory reaction. I do not imply that all early abortions are caused by bacteria; I imply simply that all such fetuses which have been examined have been associated with massive bacterial invasion.

Four- to Six-Month Abortion

During the four- to six-month period there are three major types of abortion: (1) twins; (2) definite bacterial septicemias (22); and (3) undetermined.

Group 1, twins, is discussed below.

Group 2 is a small group. The fetus is obviously septicemic with a yellowish-red, dirty discoloration of the tissues, and petechial hemorrhages on any or all serosal surfaces. There may be intense hyperemia of the mucosa of the gastrointestinal tract, the lungs, spleen, and other organs. There is no evidence of decomposition. Pure cultures of one of the several accepted abortifacient pathogens may be obtained (*Streptococcus*, *E. coli*, *C. equi*, etc.), and the histological picture is dominated by hemorrhage, intravascular bacteria, and scattered ischemic necrosis in the several parenchymal organs.

Group 3, the largest group, are those fetuses with varying degrees of decomposition. The outstanding hallmark of decomposition in the fetus is yellow-red, muddy discoloration of all tissues—precisely as described for the septic fetus. With advanced decomposition there is no problem; the liver is mushy, the abdominal viscera are muddy and blurred in appearance, and there is dirty, red-tinged fluid in the abdominal and thoracic cavities. With lesser degrees of decomposition, however, only the yellowish-red muddy appearance may be present and the prosector is on the horns of a dilemma: rot only, or rot plus septicemia. The results of bacteriological examination may be negative, hopelessly mixed, or a pure culture of an acceptable pathogen. In the latter case, one should like to see relevant histological changes. The decomposed state of the tissues, however, renders histological study not only difficult but often impossible. The fetus is not yet capable of an inflammatory reaction, ischemic necrosis is obscured by rot, and the intravascular bacteria are either not present, not observed, or if observed possibly postmortem in origin.

In this situation the diagnosis of abortion caused by bacterial septicemia is based entirely on the isolation of an accepted pathogenic organism, primarily a streptococcus. I am, frankly, miserably unhappy with this situation. It is both possible and probable that the ubiquitous streptococcus can invade a fetus and/or placenta lying dead in the uterus with the cervix dilating in preparation for abortion. It is known that streptococci and, indeed, a variety of organisms can enter the uterus whenever the cervix is open. It is also known that the fetus is dead for some time before abortion occurs, and thus the two requisite conditions for postmortem bacterial invasion are established.

It is my opinion, therefore, that the cause of most four- to six-month decomposed abortions is undetermined. In a number of instances, there is a history of the mare being ill for any one of a variety of reasons three to four days or more before the abortion. One may argue that the death of the fetus and preparation for abortion are the cause of the illness, and the argument is a cogent one. Until it is proven, however, it should be remembered that primary illness of the mare could result, secondarily, in death and abortion of the fetus.

Since the second wave of corpora lutea are waning and the maintenance of pregnancy is being taken over by the placenta or some other extraovarian source of progesterone during this four- to six-month period, it may be suggested that an upset in the transference of endocrine responsibility is involved.

Six- to Eleven-Month Abortion

From six to eleven months the pathologist has the best opportunity to clearly determine the cause of abortion. Decomposed fetuses of the undetermined type do occur sporadically throughout this period. Septicemic fetuses are aborted in reasonably fresh condition with the lesions described above. Also, the allantochorion may show splashes of hemorrhage on the chorial surface because of bacterial infection of the allantochorion as well as the fetus. Over the years various organisms have been isolated (22). With the unexplained disappearance of *Salmonella abortus-equi* none of these bacterial agents represents an epizootic problem—purely a single mare problem.

During the early part of the six- to eleven-month period hyperemia, hemorrhage, ischemic necrosis, and intra- and extravascular accumulations of bacteria are seen histologically. Toward the end of the period, eight to eleven months, light inflammatory cell reactions appear as the fetus acquires defensive competency.

Mycotic infections are a delight (1, 63). They produce marked, striking lesions and are readily diagnosed. The great majority of infections cause severe ulcerations and necrosis of the chorial surface of the allantochorion in the area of the cervical seal. The chorial lesion is sharply bounded by a hemorrhagic border and consists of yellow-brown necrosis, denudation, and ulceration (Fig. 98). A variable quantity of thick, viscid, tenacious, gray-yellow exudate is adherent to the involved area. This exudate varies from barely perceptible to a voluminous, sticky mass.

I have seen only one case of invasion of the fetal lungs by fungus and no example of skin infection. If lesions are present elsewhere on the allantochorion, the major lesion is always present in the cervical area. Rarely, the fungus may in some unexplained way invade only the amnion, producing severe, discrete, necrotic lesions.

Aspergillus sp. has been isolated or identified microscopically most frequently but mixed infections with *Mucor*, *Aspergillus*, and a variety of bacteria (the bacteriologist never sorted them out) may occur.

The lesions described are typical of mycotic placentitis but they are not, unfortunately, restricted to mycotic placentitis. Either streptococci or a mixed bacterial flora may, on occasion, be associated with precisely the same lesions. Histological and bacteriological studies must be carried out in support of the gross diagnosis.

It may be of interest to digress at this point and consider the mode of infection. The specific organism causing necrotizing placentitis is of really no moment whatsoever, whether fungus or bacteria or both. The basic, and not understood, pathological process is of considerably more interest and importance. Clinicians have observed on numerous occasions that the cervix of the mare may dilate and close again at any time during the last three or four months of pregnancy. Colonel Sager remarked that he was extremely startled when examining a mare with the speculum in the last part of pregnancy to see the foal look out at him as through a window! The speculum

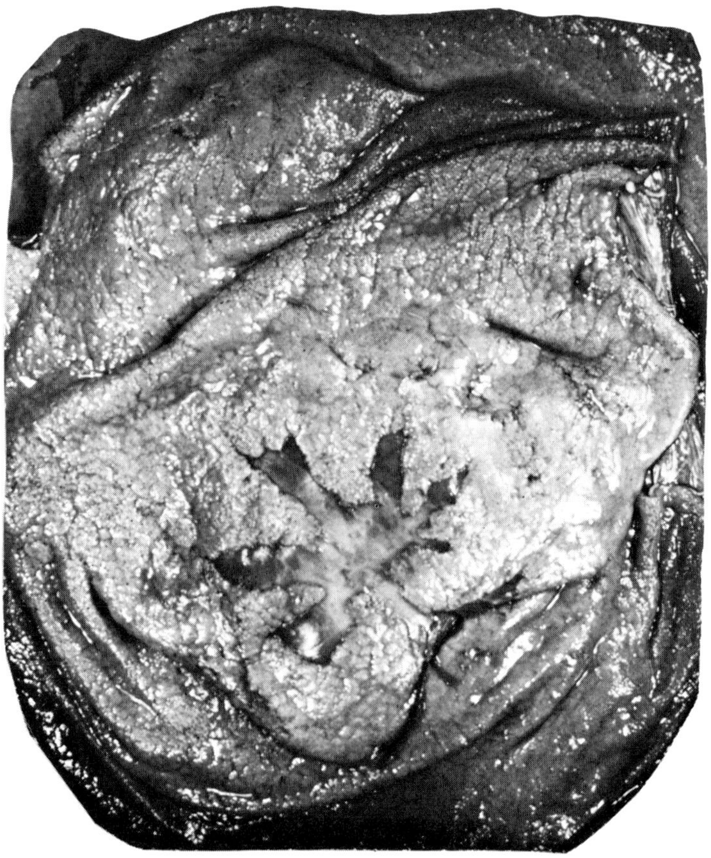

FIG. 98. Necrosis around the cervical seal of the allantochorion caused by *Aspergillus* spp. (mycotic placentitis).

was hastily withdrawn, and the mare went to term normally.

The cause of such cervical "pulsation" is surely unknown at the present time, but it may be normal or at least not a serious pathological phenomenon—not serious, that is, if the cervix closes again before bacteria or fungi are aspirated into the vagina and onto the placental membranes stretched across the open cervix.

It has been assumed for years that infection entered the uterus only at the time of breeding. It is much more reasonable, however, that the responsible organism enters only a short time before abortion. It is difficult to conceive of fungi or bacteria lying dormant in the uterus for eight months and suddenly invading and causing abortion. Perhaps, then, the major point of investigation should be the normal mechanisms and misadventures of the cervix in the pregnant mare. If it opens, the specific organism which enters the uterus is of very little moment.

We may now press on to placental diseases, "nondescriptus." While what has been said above may have been confusing, what comes next is infinitely worse. One can with sufficient work clearly differentiate bacterial and mycotic placentitis. Further, it is my belief that one can clearly distinguish a fetus which has been aborted as a result of a chronically inadequately functioning placenta. The difficulty lies in determining what, precisely, is wrong with that inadequately functioning placenta and what is the cause (74).

The fetus, usually fresh, is smaller than normal for the time of gestation, and clearly emaciated. The tissues and organs have a blanched, pale, pastel coloration rather than deep, rich, normal colors. The liver may be somewhat or considerably larger than normal and distinctly discolored. Rather than a tan to mahogany color the liver has a focal or diffuse yellowish, gray, or, in extreme cases, clay-yellow color (Fig. 99). One should not mistake pale tan rib impressions for this change. Minute white foci are extramedullary hematopoietic foci.

The color changes described are the result of uneven blood distribution, loss of glycogen, fatty metamorphosis, vacuolar degeneration, sinusoidal lining cell proliferation, and diffuse necrosis (infrequent). This description fits twins as well, being a type of placental disease, as shall be discussed below.

The gross appearance of the placenta varies over a wide range. Although one can often determine that there is a placental lesion, it is rare that one can with certainty decide the cause of the lesion. Some allantochorions simply have a marked paucity of villi, and it is clear that the fetus was chronically malnourished because of lack of metabolic exchange surface. No cause for such poor placentation has been found, and one may have to turn to "congenital malformation of the placenta" or villous hypoplasia as a diagnostic term.

A distinct lesion, body pregnancy, is occasionally seen (Fig. 100). Apparently the fetus develops in the body of the uterus, and the horns of the placenta never develop. Abortion occurs, presumably, when the fetal requirement for nutrients exceeds

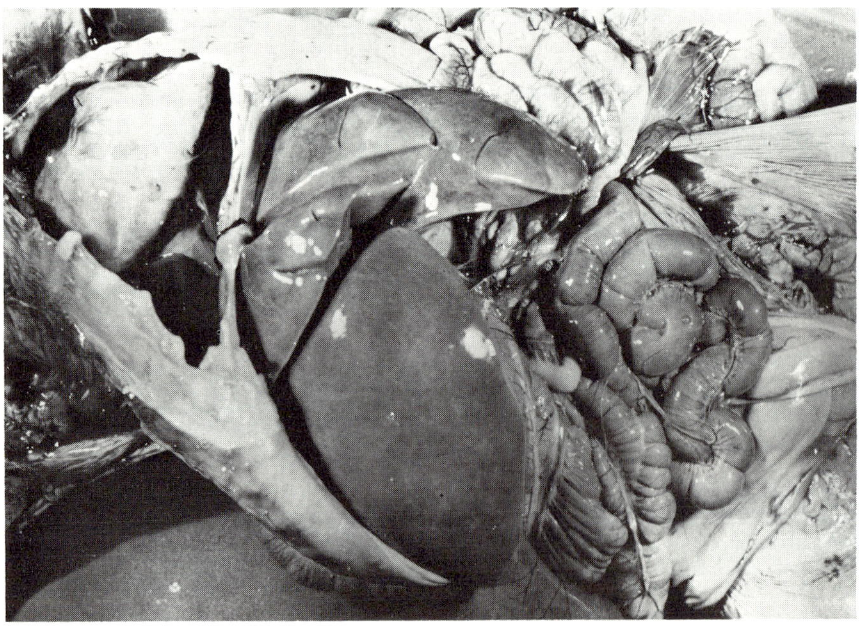

FIG. 99. Placental disease, "malnourished" fetus. The thorax is to the left of the picture. The liver is larger in the fetus than in the postnatal animal, but not as large as is seen with placental disease.

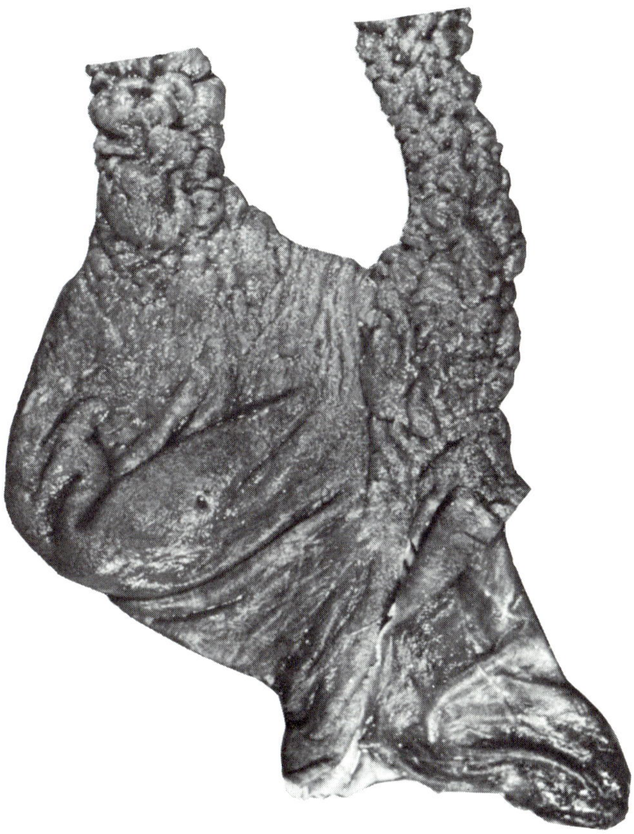

FIG. 100. "Body pregnancy" placenta. The body is large while the horns are small and deeply corrugated.

the exchange surface of the placenta. The cause of this malformation is not known.

One may see infarction of the amnion with large pale-white areas surrounded by hemorrhagic borders. Microscopically, thrombi of unknown etiology have been found in the arteries. Rarely, the amnion may be thickened and have an intensely green color. The microscopic picture is one of intense inflammation with numerous neutrophiles. No organisms have been isolated.

Many placentas have no gross changes or only irregular, variable degrees of color change on the chorial surface. The placenta comes under suspicion because of the characteristic changes in the fetus. Microscopic examination reveals a variety of changes which, at the present time, cannot be clearly classified. There may be perivascular foci of mononuclear cell infiltration, suggesting an allergic or immune process. Often there is simply fibrosis of villi, nonspecific necrosis of small blood vessels in the villi, hyalinization of the connective tissue stroma, necrosis of individual villi, fusion of villi, etc. These changes are generally focal and irregular in distribution, often obscured by postmortem changes, and difficult to interpret since all such changes occur as part of the normal placental aging process.

Chronic inflammatory lesions are occasionally seen. It appears that the placenta was infected and successfully defended itself. The attendant loss of nutrient exchange surface, however, leads to eventual malnourishment and abortion of the fetus (Fig. 101).

Microscopic calcification is common in the allantochorion and may be either antemortem or postmortem. Antemortem calcification is dystrophic; that is, it occurs in necrotic and dying tissues. Postmortem calcification is more diffuse than antemortem and often appears as plugs in the placental blood vessels.

When obviously malnourished fetuses are not accompanied by gross or microscopic placental lesions, it may be suggested that there are either functional or anatomical lesions of the endometrium or the endometrial-chorial interface. In other words malnourishment of the fetus may be the fault of the mare entirely. As discussed earlier, anatomical changes in the endometrium are not startling. The increase of endometrial atrophy and cyst formation with age is not paralleled, in my experience, by an increase in nonspecific placental disease. In short, while posing yet another possibility, I am unable on morphological grounds to substantiate that possibility.

Premature separation of the allantochorion from the endometrium does occur and cause or accompany abortion. If examined in the fresh state, immediately after abortion, the chorial surface has variably sized areas (often the entire pregnant horn) of

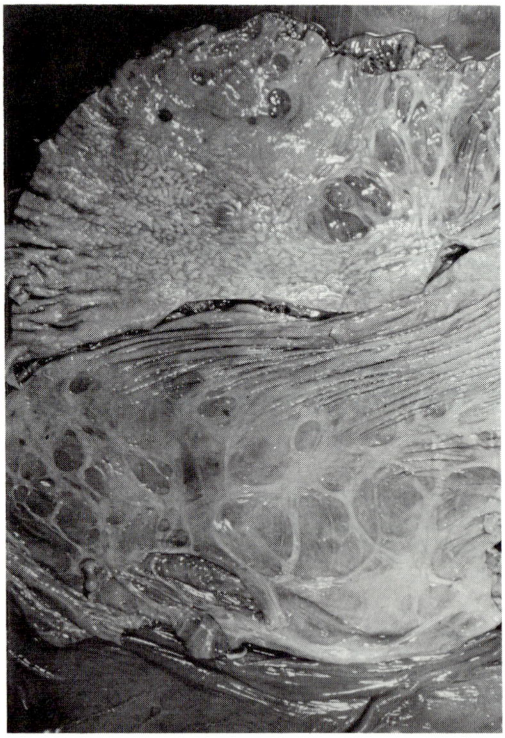

FIG. 101. Marked scarring of the allantoic surface—chronic placentitis. The normal, smooth allantoic surface is apparent at the very bottom of the picture.

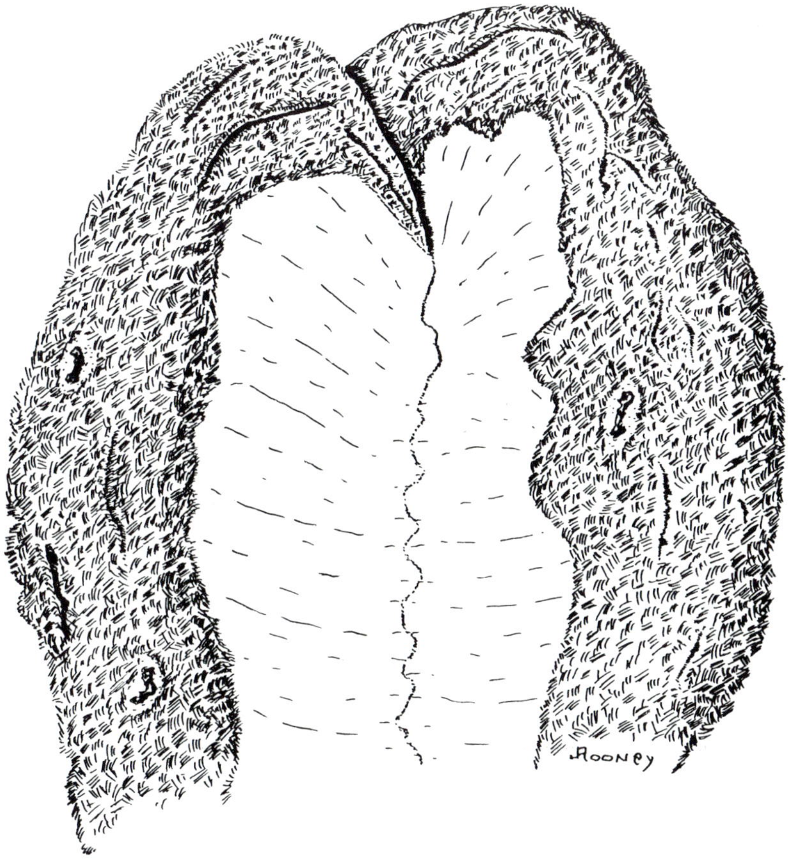

FIG. 102. Twin allantochorions with absence of villi where they were in apposition. Small bare areas with necrotic centers have also been represented. They are common in the placenta and have no pathological significance.

dry, brownish-tan discoloration, indicating death and separation of the allantochorion. No cause for the separation has been discovered, but it is clear that such separations are real and either cause or, at least, accompany abortion.

There are a number of "normal" lesions of the placenta which need to be distinguished from significant lesions. The cervical area of the allantochorion is normally devoid of villi and has irregular gray thickenings and hyperemic patches. Small 0.1- to 1.0-cm. bare areas may be scattered over the chorial surface. They often have raised, irregular brownish centers which may be calcified (Fig. 102). The blood content of the allantochorion is variable and may be deep-red in one area, pale in another, and intensely hyperemic in another. The normal term placenta has a small quantity of brownish-red exudate on the chorial surface.

The allantoic surface may be smooth and unremarkable or have one or many polypoid white masses of varying size. These are hippomanes. The common, oval, olive-green hippomane apparently arises from these polypoid masses by increasing in mass, pedicle formation, necrosis, and separation from the pedicle. Occasionally, there are small areas of folding of the allantochorion with two chorial surfaces pressed firmly together. The fold can be pulled out, revealing chorial surfaces completely devoid of villi. These are of no pathological significance (see discussion of twins, below).

The surface of the umbilical cord may be studded with calcified plaques, polyps, and, occasionally, a large pedunculated ball composed of plates of calcium or coarse-fiber bone. These are of the same nature as hippomanes and should not be confused with twinning.

The twisted umbilical cord has been frequently incriminated as a cause of abortion; this is sheer nonsense. The umbilical cord is normally markedly twisted and the postmortem pooling of blood provides a variable picture of hyperemia. Rarely the cord may be wrapped around the head of the fetus or around a leg with severe edema and passive hyperemia evident in both the cord and the fetal part.

The normal, term placenta contracts remarkably after parturition, squeezing blood from the placenta into the foal. The inexperienced prosector may be quite startled by the small size of the allantochorion as compared to the foal once this contraction has been completed.

Twin pregnancy is pathological and quite common in the mare. Although rhinopneumonitis might have a percentage lead in any given year, the main cause of abortion in Thoroughbred and Standardbred mares, over a period of years, is twinning. As a rule one twin will be dead and rotten (and/or mummified) and the other will be smaller than normal and show the placental disease, malnutrition lesions described above. On occasion both twins appear to have been alive at the time of abortion. Abortion may occur at any time during pregnancy.

The fetal membranes are characteristic even if only one twin is submitted for examination (the small, macerated fetus is often overlooked or mashed into the straw by the mare). The two allantochorions press against each other, preventing normal villus formation, and thereby depriving the fetuses of nutrient exchange surface (Fig. 102).

I have only seen one definite example of identical twinning in mares (of some 600 such abortions examined); there were two amniotic sacs and a single allantochorion (Fig. 103).

Malformations as a cause of fetal abortion are rare. Such malformations as do occur (contracted foals, blindness, cardiac anomalies, etc.) do not as a rule result in abortion. An occasional contracted foal may be so malformed that the abdomen

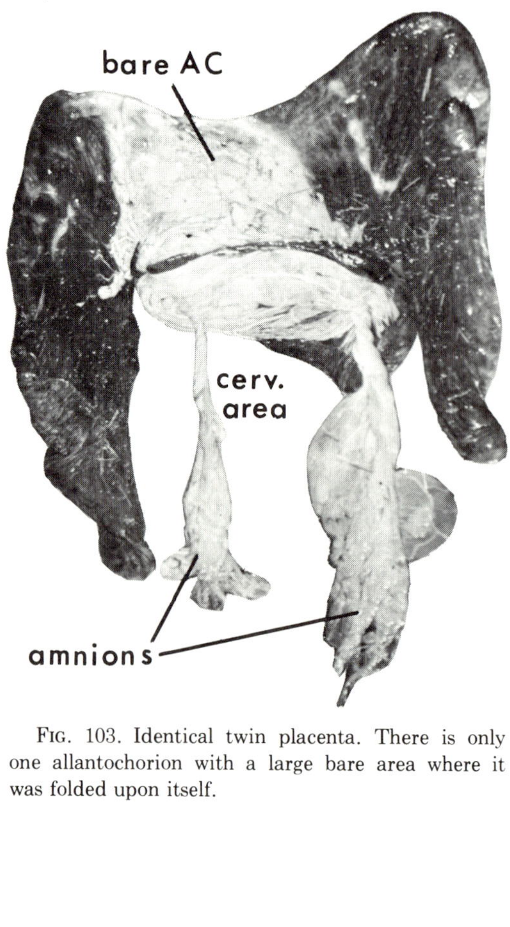

FIG. 103. Identical twin placenta. There is only one allantochorion with a large bare area where it was folded upon itself.

fails to close (73) and death and abortion follow.

Many aborted fetuses have a "frosting" of lacy, whitish granular material adherent to the skin. This is crystalline material precipitated from the amniotic fluid and is of no known pathological significance.

One fetus had massive, virtually complete calcification of both lungs. Several cases of severe mononuclear, giant cell pneumonia have been seen in fetuses during the six- to eleven-month period. There has been one case of giant cell hepatitis. Marked enlargement of the thyroids (colloid goiter, histologically) and persistence of the thyroglossal duct have been seen with some frequency in aborted fetuses and newborn foals (see p. 103). In none of these cases (except goiter) has the cause been determined.

Rhinopneumonitis has been well described (26, 65), and it will only be necessary for us to consider the gross autopsy findings. The typical case is aborted quickly, without premonitory signs and in fresh condition. It seems clear that in most cases the fetus is alive when the process of abortion begins.

There is fetal diarrhea (asphyxia; see below) with greenish, meconium staining of both the amnion and the fetus. The mucous membranes of the eyes and mouth may have multiple fine petechiae. There may be subcutaneous edema over the nose and forehead. The subcutaneous tissues of the axillary and femoral areas contain yellowish edema. The pleural cavity contains a variable quantity of clear, straw-colored fluid (Fig. 104). The mediastinal tissues are yellow and edematous. There are multiple fine epicardial and endocardial petechiae and variable but usually prominent bands of interlobular edema in the lungs with petechial pleural hemorrhages. The lungs are heavier than normal. There are variably severe hemorrhages in the trachea, the tissues of the thoracic inlet, and elsewhere in the body. Fluid is normally present in the guttural pouches of the aborted fetus and should not be considered part of the disease process. The liver has multiple, fine white foci of necrosis in about 10% of the cases. The spleen is swollen and dark-red on section. The mesenteric lymph nodes and the root of the mesentery are edematous as are the tissues in the portal area of the liver.

This is the classical, full-blown case of rhinopneumonitis. Obviously, one does not see all these lesions in every case. The lesions may be present in full or only in part and the degree of change in any one part can vary widely. Disturbingly, an occasional rotten fetus may, microscopically, have characteristic lesions of rhinopneumonitis. The gross positive diagnosis, then, is rarely incorrect, but a gross negative diagnosis may be incorrect.

There are no placental lesions with rhinopneumonitis, but the virus can be the immediate cause of abortion in fetuses already affected by more chronic problems such as twinning, body pregnancy, mycotic placentitis, etc.

The causes of abortion have been summarized in Tables 2 and 3. Table 3 represents experience and opinion and is in no sense to be taken as precise quantitative data. There will be considerable variation from year to year, and the percentage figures represent only the relative incidence of the several types of abortion.

Term Foal

The term foal presents interesting problems of transition from intra- to extrauterine life. We shall be concerned here with some few facts and speculations about the failure to make that transition. The causes of death in this period may be broadly

TABLE 2

Time of Abortion	Causes
Early	Infection, unknown
4 to 6 months	Unknown, twins, fetal infection, placental disease
6 to 11 months	Twins, virus, placental disease, fetal infection, unknown

TABLE 3

Type of Abortion	Incidence %
Rhinopneumonitis abortion	10
Twins	20
Fetal infection (bacterial)	10
Bacterial-mycotic placentitis	10
Placental malformations*	10
Miscellaneous (hepatitis, congenital malformation, etc.)	2
Unknown	38
Total	100

* Defined pathologically as abnormal but cause unknown.

grouped into (1) neonatal asphyxia, and (2) prematurity.

Neonatal Asphyxia. For the postmortem diagnosis of neonatal asphyxia one first ascertains a general set of lesions, and then attempts to determine the specific cause of the general lesions in that particular case.

The general set of lesions is petechiation of the mucosae of eyes, mouth, trachea and bronchi, epicardium, and endocardium. There is edema of the root of the mesentery and the portal area of the liver (the latter two lesions are highly characteristic). The lungs may be completely atelectatic, partially aerated, or fully aerated. In other words, the foal may or may not breathe during or after delivery. The lesions obviously are those of asphyxiation.

Delayed delivery is the most common specific cause of neonatal asphyxia. Such delay may be caused by an overly large foal in a small mare. More often a malposition of the foal at the time of delivery causes the delay. The allantochorion separates in due course, and if the foal is not delivered promptly, it will not receive oxygen either from the mare or from the air.

There is, of course, a bewildering variety of such malpositions, but this is not our present concern. The caudal or breech presentation is quite dangerous. Since the cord is attached near the caudal end of the foal, it will be compressed in the pelvis early in the course of delivery. Under these circumstances even rapid delivery may not be rapid enough. Malformations are, as a cause of dystocia, simply a special case of malposition.

Delayed delivery neonatal asphyxia can be very unsettling for the inexperienced pathologist and for those responsible for the foal. More often than not the foal will be submitted with no history, or with one that reports, "She delivered with no trouble with me standing right there!" The autopsy reveals no specific lesions, only neonatal asphyxia, and the prosector wonders where he has failed. There may be bruising or even separation at the costochondral junctions, but this is common and unimportant. Open the shoulder joints. If the synovial fluid is bloody and the articular cartilages are stained with blood, a diagnosis of delayed delivery can be made. The foal was delayed and squeezed in the pelvic canal. (I do not know whether there is blood in the shoulder joints of some, or all, normal foals born at term. I do know that no foal which has lived 12–24 hours or so has such bleeding, and the cartilage staining is unlikely to clear in that short a time.) The simple maneuver of opening the shoulder joint and exclaiming, "This foal didn't get out in time!" will frequently cause the groom or attendant to admit that it had not indeed been delivered in time, or that he was not in reality in attendance at the time of foaling. He may try to intimate that he was only away for two minutes for a smoke or coffee, and it is probably best to appear to agree—and mark "neonatal asphyxia, delayed delivery" on your protocol.

When an owner or inexperienced manager submits the foal, he will rarely know just what did happen (even if he witnessed the foaling) and will always be at some

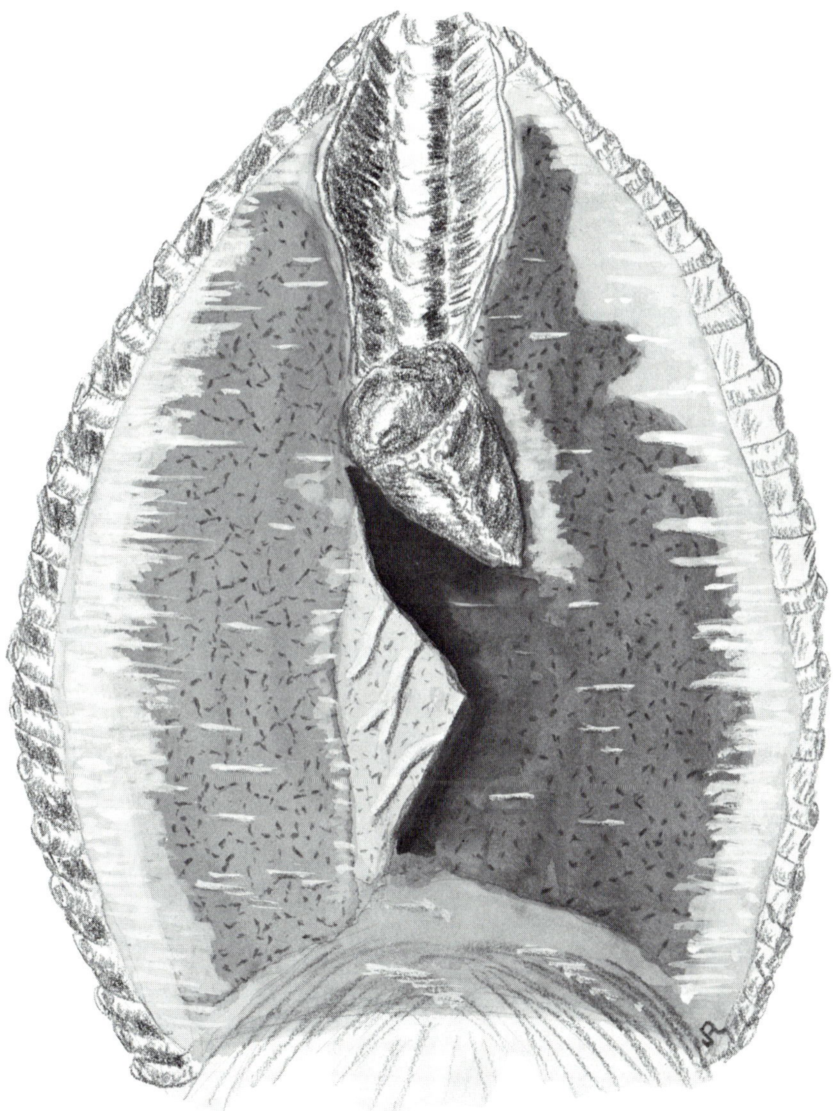

FIG. 104. Pleural effusion characteristic of fetal rhinopneumonitis.

pains to conceal or deny any evidence of improper management or ignorance on his part. He may fire the night watchman when he gets home, but he won't tell the prosector.

The foal may be traumatized as a result of malposition or malformation either because of the effort of the mare or man to effect delivery. The major traumatic lesion is fractured ribs. These fractures occur near the middle third and are to be distinguished from the common, quite insignificant, costochondral separations mentioned earlier. Such rib fractures may be clinically unimportant, or they may puncture and scarify the heart and/or lungs and result in significant hemorrhage and death.

Maiden mares may panic and race about the stall swinging the half-delivered foal behind them, inflicting a variety of injuries. Maiden mares also may refuse to lie down for delivery, thus in some unknown mannner delaying delivery.

The weak foal which reaches term with a mycotic or bacterial placentitis may not have sufficient reserves to withstand even the short period of asphyxia during pelvic delivery.

Those foals which show evidence of acute septicemia at birth or within the first few hours of life probably acquired that infection *in utero* or during delivery. Most such infections are caused by *Shigella* or *E. coli* from contaminated urine or feces aspirated into the vagina and uterus once the cervix has opened. Incidentally, as is discussed below, some of these early septicemias may present with so-called "barker foal" clinical signs.

There are two types of improper placental separation which result in neonatal asphyxia. The first and most obvious is when, for some unknown reason, the body of the placenta breaks off near the middle instead of at the cervical seal area as it normally should. A large portion of the allantochorion is then delivered before the amniotic sac or the foal appears. Unless delivered rapidly such foals die of asphyxiation.

The second type of separation is considerably less obvious. Careful examination of the allantochorion of the asphyxiated foal may show that the body and/or part of the gravid horn had been separating for some time before labor began. The normal chorial surface is velvety in texture and a deep, rich, red color. With premature separation the affected part of the allantochorion will be slightly drier and tan in color. This determination must only be made on the placenta delivered immediately or very shortly after the foal. If delivery of the placenta is delayed for an hour or more, the entire chorial surface will show this tan, "dying" color, and no conclusions can be drawn. Since, in the case of premature separation of this type, most of the allantochorion will be separated at the time of foaling, it will as a rule be delivered quickly and the diagnosis can be made.

Neither of these two types of placental separation is common (2–3 cases/100 neonatal deaths/year), and the cause is not known.

Next we come to the vexing condition known as "barker foal." These foals are born normally and expeditiously and develop an apparent convulsive air hunger within a few hours after birth. Many so-called barker foals in my Kentucky experience were, in fact, septicemic foals afflicted with *E. coli* or *Shigella*.

Most reports of barker foal have come from England and Ireland, and much has been made of this geographical distribution. I have had the opportunity to examine sections of lung and a few other tissues from eleven cases of the series on which the original published description

(64) was based. Rather than the reported atelectasis, there were histological changes of septicemia and/or bacterial pneumonia in six cases. The other five cases had histories at least suggestive of neonatal asphyxia, although no microscopic lesions could be found in the tissues available. I do not contend that there is no such entity as the barker foal; it is simply that I have not personally seen a case that could not be better explained on the basis of the available pathological evidence.

One occasionally finds rupture of the liver (usually middle lobe) in the newborn foal or aborted fetus. In both cases insufficient dilatation of the cervix is probably the important factor. As the cause of death in the term foal, ruptured liver is usually associated with other lesions, such as fractured ribs, shoulder joint hemorrhage, etc. Liver rupture in the aborted fetus is incidental and should not be mistaken for the cause of abortion.

Premature Foal. The premature foal is a vexing problem not infrequently thrown into the lap of the pathologist: "This foal was weak when it was born and only lived a few hours (or days). Is it premature?" The pathologist can determine the immediate cause of death in most cases (a septicemia or pneumonia), but the question of prematurity remains open. The only lesion which I have been able to associate with prematurity is a gas-filled small intestine and large intestine, particularly the former. Obviously, this "lesion" can only be determined immediately after death, before decomposition sets in. I have never been able to associate respiratory problems, so common in the comparable human situation, with prematurity in the foal. If delivered more than a week or two before the proper foaling date, most foals will die sooner or later, and usually sooner. The only assistance that can be offered at this time is the gaseous small intestine, without even a hypothesis to explain that.

Young Foals

The many and varied conditions which affect young foals have been discussed throughout the book. We may summarize some of the more important points at this time.

The major causes of illness and death in young foals are bacterial and parasitic disease followed by hemolytic icterus and a miscellaneous variety of viral, mycotic, and traumatic events.

During the first two weeks of life septicemia caused by *Shigella equi* infection is a major problem. Age resistance quickly develops, however, and fatal disease beyond the first month is uncommon. The autopsy picture is dominated by dirty, yellowish discoloration of all tissues, acute synovitis, perirenal edema, multiple renal cortical abscesses (purulent glomeruli), and a distinct sewage-type odor when the carcass is opened. Broad spectrum antibiotics, administered after prompt diagnosis, have reduced the mortality almost to zero. Too often, however, the first clinical signs are misinterpreted. The foal may simply show pain (lameness) in one leg and stop nursing. The horseman thinks the mare kicked it and waits. The acute synovitis worsens, the septicemia is overwhelming, and the foal is in shock (semicomatose, "sleeper") before the error becomes apparent. Even heroic therapy will often fail at this late stage. Any illness or slight change in behavior of any sort during the first month of life should be considered shigellosis until proven otherwise.

E. coli septicemia also occurs during the first week, and causes a violent clinical disease very similar to *Shigella* infection. Severe diarrhea and shock quickly lead to a fatal outcome. Therapy has not often been successful, and it is fortunate that *E. coli* septicemia is not common. At autopsy the lesions are identical to those seen with shigellosis with the exception of renal cortical abscessation.

Streptococci are a major cause of septicemia in foals during the first two to three months. Foals infected at birth or during the first week have clinical signs and course similar to shigellosis. The synovitis is often more purulent in character, however. With increasing age the clinical course is more prolonged, and purulent umbilicus-urachus, joint, and lung involvement are more prominent.

Ascarid infestation and bloodworm infestation kill or maim many young foals every year. Heavy ascarid infestations can cause perforation of the small intestine and fatal peritonitis. Somewhat lesser degrees of infestation cause diarrhea, are debilitating, and may cause ileus with subsequent intussusception, volvulus, etc.

Young foals, with their curious eating habits, can acquire heavy bloodworm infestations. There have been a number of cases of thromboembolic infarction of the large intestine in foals 29 to 30 days of age. Since the larvae reach the ileocecocolic artery about three weeks after ingestion, it is apparent that the foal acquired the larvae during the first week of life. There is no evidence of intrauterine transmission.

Hemolytic icterus is a common and well known condition in the neonate. The autopsy findings are clear: severe anemia and variable degrees of icterus. An excellent recent review is available (25, 45).

Thus concludes our discussion of fetal and neonatal disease. Many questions remain open; there are very few clear answers. What has been attempted, as throughout this book, is a presentation of the results of my experience. While my experience has been unique and extensive in the area of fetal and neonatal disease of the horse, it provides only a starting point for many more observations and research.

TWELVE

Special Examinations and Recording

Special Examinations

Having completed a careful, systematic gross examination, the prosector must evaluate his findings in relation to the clinical history and determine the additional examinations or studies required to establish a diagnosis.

At this point the factual training and interpretative abilities of the prosector receive a severe test. Lack of confidence or knowledge may lead to a welter of tests which reflect only the prosector's desperate desire to cover any and all possibilities. If any basic rule can be applied to aid the prosector, it must be that the best diagnosis is an etiological diagnosis. One should always be alert to the possibility of multiple eitology (bacteria and virus; trauma and predisposing structural defects).

Special examinations are: (1) bacteriological, virological, serological; (2) parasitological; (3) chemical and biochemical; (4) roentgenological; and (5) histological.

Bacteriology, Virology, and Serology

As a general rule any local pathological changes which may be infectious in nature are submitted for examination: abscesses, phlegmons, pericardial, pleural, peritoneal exudates, consolidated lung, etc. If the gross examination indicates septicemia, the examination of focal lesions must be supplemented by study of the regional lymph nodes, nonregional lymph nodes, spleen, and heart blood. In septicemias of enteric origin the intestine, mesenteric lymph nodes, liver, spleen, heart blood, and one or more other lymph nodes should be examined.

Frequently, the autopsy will not uncover specific lesions which cry for further study. Diseases involving the central nervous system, for example, are often not accompanied by characteristic gross lesions. The clinical history, if properly taken and properly evaluated, will help the prosector to decide which require bacteriological and/or virological examination.

No matter what materials are selected for examination the prosector must adhere to the following precepts:

1. Bacteriological and virological samples must be collected and handled in as aseptic a manner as possible.
2. A resumé of the clinical history and gross findings together with the autopsy diagnosis (or differential diagnoses) should be provided for the guidance of the microbiologist.

Ideally, materials for bacteriological or virological study should be delivered immediately to the appropriate laboratory. If, as is often the case under field conditions, immediate delivery is impossible, the samples should be placed in clean (preferably sterile) bottles or plastic bags and shipped frozen in abundant quantity of Dry Ice or water ice. The fastest available transportation should be employed.

Blood samples collected for serological study should be allowed to clot on the slant; the serum should be poured off and the sample shipped under refrigeration or frozen in tightly stoppered or screw-cap vials. Whole blood should not be frozen.

Parasitology

Ectoparasites or skin lesions suspected to be of parasitic or mycotic origin should be subjected to laboratory examination. The parasites themselves or deep, adequate scrapings of suspected lesions may be examined directly, given to the parasitologist, or preserved in 70% alcohol for shipment. In many cases it is preferable to submit a tissue specimen fresh or with one-half fixed for histology and the other half fresh for culture.

Gastrointestinal contents are spread out, diluted if necessary, in glass dishes and examined for the presence of parasites. Specimens for further identification may be preserved in 70% alcohol. Protozoa, of course, cannot be seen with the naked eye and microscopic examination is necessary. If blood parasites (*Piroplasma*, for example) are suspected, impression smears of blood and spleen should be prepared.

Chemistry and Biochemistry

In general, tissues for chemical analysis should be generous and shipped in glass or plastic in the frozen state. Suspected poisoning cases, with the ever-present possibility of medicolegal complications, require special handling. Every effort should be made to have the autopsy performed by a qualified pathologist. All materials selected for toxicological study must be placed in sealed containers and handled so that continuous, legal possession may be established. In general, urine, bile, gastrointestinal content, liver, and kidney should be saved in cases of acute poisoning.

Roentgenology

Examinations have already been discussed.

Histology

As a general rule all lesions should be examined microscopically if their nature is not readily apparent to the naked eye. In addition, certain organs and tissues will be examined in the absence of gross lesions if the suspected disease is known to produce lesions in such organs or tissues. This presupposes, of course, familiarity with the usual site of microscopic lesions. If in doubt, sample and submit everything.

Despite many words written and spoken on the necessity for taking small pieces of tissue to include both grossly pathological, borderline, and normal tissue, most prosectors continue to attempt submission of whole organs crammed into pint jars (or smaller!).

Recording the Findings

The art of describing the autopsy findings in detail is as important as making the post mortem dissection. One is forced to do good work and learn to make understandable observations, and the observations are preserved for the future.

All deviations from the normal should first be written down without discussion of the nature of origin of the changes. Carl Rokitansky (1804–1878), pathologist of Vienna, and considered to be the greatest descriptive pathologist of all time, formulated the basic precepts for the description of all lesions: size, shape, position, color, consistency, cut surface.

Lesions encountered during the course of the external examination as well as during the evisceration and examination of the organs should be carefully described. A diagnosis is not a description! Do not record: "A large abscess in the left flank." Do record: "A 15- by 20-cm. well encapsulated abscess was present in the subcutaneous tissue in the dorsal third of the paralumbar area. The content was dry and caseous in nature with a distinct olive-green color. The abscess wall was 1 cm. thick and composed of white, firm tissue. Upon removal of the content the inner surface of the capsule appeared ragged with numerous tags of dirty brown tissue hanging into the abscess cavity."

The intensity of the lesions should be recorded; perhaps as follows: (1) normal; (2) slight (questionable, may or may not be a lesion); (3) mild (definite change); (4) moderate; (5) marked; and (6) severe.

The size and extent of a lesion should, at best, be described by metric measurement: 20 by 15 mm., 3 by 8 cm., etc. However, I do feel that there are mitigating circumstances. Often such precision is meaningless. The prosector is simply not going to measure petechiae with a millimeter rule or evacuate every cyst and measure the contents (how much lost in transfer?). Often a reasonable approximation is better than meaningless precision.

When all examinations have been completed, one should review the descriptions of the findings and prepare a list of diagnoses. This list should be as much as possible in order of importance, showing the chronology of the disease processes. Finally, a pathological-anatomical diagnosis, at best an etiological diagnosis, is synthesized from the list.

One should not simply prepare a list rigidly and blindly. The real purpose of the autopsy is to reveal and relate the course of events from the normal through the disease state to death. A brief summary of the natural history of the disease process is the desideratum.

References

1. Ainsworth, G. C. and Austwick, P. K. C. Fungal diseases of animals. *Commonw. Agric. Bur., England*, 1959.
2. Alexander, F. The rate of passage of food residues through the digestive tract of the horse. *J. Comp. Path. 56:* 266–268, 1946.
3. Alexander F. The effects of some humoral agents on the horse lleum. *Brit. J. Pharmacol. 7:* 25–32, 1952.
4. Baker, H. J. and Lindsey, J. R. Equine goiter due to excess dietary iodide. *J. Amer. Vet. Med. Ass. 153:* 1618–1630, 1968.
5. Bäriswyl, von K. and Gerber, H. Pankreasvergrösserung beim Pferd mögliche klinische Bedeutung und pathologish-anatomisches Bild. *Deutsch. Tierärztl. Wschr. 71:* 436–438, 1964.
6. Bennett, S. P. and Franco, D. A. Equine protozoan diarrhea (equine intestinal trichomoniasis) at Trinidad racetracks. *J. Amer. Vet. Med. Ass. 154:* 58–60, 1969.
7. Berge, E. Ueber die lokale Malazie der Sesambeine am Fesselgelenke des Pferdes, ein Beitrag zue Pathologie und Klinik der "Gleichbeinlähme". *Berlin. Tierärztl. Wschr. 49:* 629–633, 645–649, 1933.
8. Berliner, V. R. The physiology of reproduction in the mare. In *Equine Medicine and Surgery*, American Veterinary Medical Publications, Santa Barbara, 1963.
9. Brandt, A. J. Über Hypophysenadenome bei Hund und Pferd. *Skand. Vet. Tidskr. 59:* 875–917, 1940.
10. Bridges, C. H. and Emmons, C. W. A phycomycosis of horses caused by *Hyphomyces destruens*. *J. Amer. Vet. Med. Ass. 138:* 579–589, 1961.
11. Bridges, C. H. Phycomycosis. In *Equine Medicine and Surgery*, American Veterinary Medical Publications, Santa Barbara, 1963.
12. Bryans, J. T. Periodic ophthalmia. In *Equine Medicine and Surgery*, American Veterinary Medical Publications, Santa Barbara, 1963.
13. Bryans, J. T. Salmonellosis. In *Equine Medicine and Surgery*, American Veterinary Medical Publications, Santa Barbara, 1963.
14. Buxton, A. Salmonellosis in animals, a review. *Commonw. Agric. Bur., England*, 1957.
15. Coffman, J. R. Personal communication, 1969.
16. Cohrs, P. *Nieberle und Cohrs: Lehrbuch der speziellen pathologischen Anatomie der Haustiere*. Gustav Fischer, Jena, 1961.
17. Cole, C. R. Changes in the equine larynx associated with laryngeal hemiplegia. *Amer. J. Vet. Res. 7:* 69, 1946.
18. Cook, W. R. The clinical features of guttural pouch mycosis in the horse. *Vet. Rec. 83:* 336–345, 1968.
19. David, J. S. E. Personal communication, 1969.
20. Detwelier, D. K. and Patterson, D. F. Diseases of the blood and cardiovascular system. In *Equine Medicine and Surgery*, American Veterinary Medical Publications, Santa Barbara, 1963.
21. Dimock, W. W. and Edwards, P. R. Pathology and bacteriology of the reproductive organs of mares in relation to sterility. *Ky. Agric. Exp. Sta. Bull. 286*, 1928.
22. Dimock, W. W., Edwards, P. R. and Bruner, D. W. Infections of fetuses and foals. *Ky. Agric. Exp. Sta. Bull. 509*, 1–40, 1947.
23. Dobberstein, J. *Richtlinien für Die Sektion Der Haustiere*, Paul Parey, Berlin, 1957.
24. Dodd, D. C. White muscle disease of foals. In *Equine Medicine and Surgery*, American Veterinary Medical Publications, Santa Barbara, 1963.
25. Doll, E. R. and Hull, F. E. Observations on hemolytic icterus of newborn foals. *Cornell Vet. 41:* 14–35, 1951.
26. Doll, E. R. Viral rhinopneumonitis. In *Equine Medicine and Surgery*, American Veterinary Medical Publications, Santa Barbara, 1963.
27. Drechsler, von O. Neue Gedanken über die Ätiologie der Längsachsendrehung des grossen Colon beim Pferd. *Deutsch. Tierärztl. Wschr. 65:* 298–303, 1958.
28. Dreguss, M. S. and Lombard, L. S. *Experimental Studies in Equine Infectious Anemia*. University of Pennsylvania Press, Philadelphia, 1954.
29. Elias, H. The Tonsils of the Horse. *Amer. J. Vet. Res. 7:* 343–349, 1946.
30. Elias, H. Growth of the adrenal cortex in domesticated ungulata. *Amer. J. Vet. Res. 9:* 173–189, 1948.

31. Enigk, K. Weitere Untersuchungen zur Biologie von *Strongylus vulgaris* (Nematodes) im Wirtstiere. *Z. Tropenmed. Parasit. 2:* 523–535, 1951.
32. Enigk, K. Die Pathogenese der thrombotisch-embolischen Kolik des Pferdes. *Mschr. Prakt. Tierheilk. 3:* 65–74, 1951.
33. Enigk, K. Zur Entwiklung von *Strongylus vulgaris* (Nematodes im Wirtstier). *Z. Tropenmed. Parasit. 2:* 287–306, 1952.
34. Enigk, K. and Grittner, I. Zur Morphologie von *Strongylus vulgaris* (Nematodes). *Z. Parasitenk. 15:* 267–282, 1952.
35. Farilly, B. Personal communication, 1966.
36. Fisher, J. R. S. Provided the case cited, 1968.
37. Georg, L. K., Kaplan, W. and Camp, L. B. Equine ringworm with special reference to *Trichophyton equinum*. *Amer. J. Vet. Res. 18:* 798–810, 1957.
38. Habel, R. E. The perineum of the mare. *Cornell Vet. 43:* 247–278, 1953.
39. Hemmert-Halswick, A. Zur Pathologie der Lymphangitis epizootica des Pferdes. *Berlin Munchen Tierarztl. Wschr.* August, 13–15, 1946.
40. Hickman, J. *Veterinary Orthopaedics*. Oliver and Boyd, Edinburgh, 1964.
41. Hirose, T. and Satoh, H. Colic of the horse and autonomic-nervous disturbances—Patho-morphological investigations. *Exp. Rep. Eq. Health Lab. 4:* 151–212, 1967.
42. Hug, A. Über chronische Atembeschwerden des Pferdes. *Schweiz. Arch. Tierheilk. 79:* 211–280, 1937.
43. Hutyra, F., Marek, J. and Manninger, R. *Special Pathology and Therapeutics of the Diseases of Domestic Animals*. Vol. 3, 4th English Ed., A. Eger, Chicago, 1938.
44. Irvine, C. Panel discussion. *Proceedings of the American Association of Equine Practitioners*, 264–265, Los Angeles, 1962.
45. Jeffcott, L. B. Haemolytic disease of the new born foal. *Eq. Vet. J. 1:* 165–170, 1969.
46. Jirina, K. Über das Vorkommen der Setarien bei Pferden. *Deutsch. Tierarztl. Wschr. 66:* 439–441, 1959.
47. Jones, T. C. Equine periodic ophthalmia. *Amer. J. Vet. Res. 3:* 45–71, 1942.
48. Jones, T. C. and Maurer, F. C. Sporotrichosis in horses. *Bull. U.S. Army Med. Dept., Wash. 74:* 63–73, 1944.
49. Jones, T. C. Doll, E. R. and Bryans, J. T. The lesions of equine viral arteritis. *Cornell Vet. 48:* 52–68, 1957.
50. Jubb, K. V. R. and Kennedy, P. C. *Pathology of Domestic Animals*. Academic Press Inc., New York, 1963.
51. King, A. S. Studies on equine purpura haemorrhagica. 3. Morbid anatomy and histology. *Vet. J. 105:* 35, 1949.
52. Knudsen, O. Partial dilatation of the uterus as a cause of sterility in the mare. *Cornell Vet. 54:* 423–438, 1964.
53. Krahnert, R. Zum Magenkrebs des Pferdes. *Mh. Vet. Med. 7:* 399–404, 1952.
54. Krause, C. Zur Frage der Arteriosklerose bei Pferd, Rind und Hund. *Beitr. Path. Anat. 71:* 121–178, 1922.
55. Krook, L. and Lowe, J. E. Nutritional secondary hyperparathyroidism in the horse. *Path. Vet.*, suppl. 1, 1964.
56. Langham, R. F. and Hallman, E. T. Some observations on nephritis in horses. *Amer. J. Vet. Res. 1:* 49–52, 1940.
57. Larsson, B., Obel, N. and Åberg, B. On the biochemistry of keratinization in the matrix of the horse's hoof in normal conditions and in laminitis. *Nordisk. Vet. 8:* 761–776, 1956.
58. Lilleengen K. Hjärtmissbildningar hos djuren. *Skand. Vet. Tidskr. 24:* 493–555, 1934.
59. Littlejohn, A. Babesiasis. In *Equine Medicine and Surgery*, American Veterinary Medical Publications, Santa Barbara, 1963.
60. Looser, F. Über die Ossifikationsstörungen bei Kretinismus. *Verhl. Deutsch. Pathol. Ges. 24:* 352–360, 1929.
61. Magnusson, H. Pyaemia in foals caused by *Corynebacterium equi*. *Vet. Rec. 50:* 1459–1468, 1938.
62. Mahaffey, L. W. Fenestration of the aortic and pulmonary valves in the horse. *Vet. Rec. 70:* 415–418, 1958.
63. Mahaffey, L. W. and Adam, N. M. Abortions associated with mycotic lesions of the placenta in mares. *J. Amer. Vet. Med. Ass. 144:* 24–32, 1964.
64. Mahaffey, L. W. and Rossdale, P. D. Convulsive and allied syndromes in new-born foals. *Vet. Rec. 69:* 1277–1286, 1957.
65. Manninger, R. and Csontos, J. Virusabortus der Stuten. *Deutsch. Tierarztl. Wschr. 49:* 105–108, 1941.
66. McFeely, R. D. and Peterson, F. In *Proceedings of the American Association of Equine Practitioners*, Houston, 1969.
67. Mollmann, L. H. Zur Pathologie des sympathischen Bauchgangliones des Pferdes—ganglion coeliacum plus mesentericum anterius—zugleich ein Beitrag zur Pathogenese der Kolik. *Z. Veterinärk. 44:* 273–288, 1932.
68. Nielsen, S. W. and Spratling, F. R. Tuberculous spondylitis in a horse. *Brit. Vet. J. 124:* 503–508, 1968.
69. Nienhaus, H. Verknöcherung der rechten Herzvorkammerwand eines Pferdes. *Deutsch. Tierarztl. Wschr. 33:* 854–855, 1925.
70. Nilsson, S. A. Bidrag till kannedomen om fotens innervation hos häst. *Skand. Vet. Tidskr. 38:* 401–460, 1948.
71. Obel, N. *Studies on the Histopathology of Acute Laminitis*. Almqvist and Wiksells, Uppsala, 1948.
72. Ottaway, C. W. and Worden, A. N. Bursae and

tendon sheaths of the horse. *Vet. Rec. 52:* 477–483, 1940.

73. Poynter, D. The arterial lesions produced by *Strongylus vulgaris* and their relationship to the migratory route of the parasite in its host. *Res. Vet. Sci. 1:* 205–217, 1960.
74. Prickett, M. E. The pathology of the equine placenta and its effects on the fetus. *Proceedings of the American Association of Equine Practitioners*, 201–214, 1967.
75. Rooney, J. R. Contracted foal. *Cornell Vet. 56:* 172–187, 1966.
76. Rooney, J. R. and Prickett, M. E. Shaker foal. *Mod. Vet. Pract. 48:* 44–45, 1967.
77. Rooney, J. R., Bryans, J. T., Prickett, M. E. and Zent, W. W. Exhaustion shock in the horse. *Cornell Vet. 56:* 220–235, 1965.
78. Rooney, J. R., Delaney, F. M. and Mayo, J. Sacroiliac luxation in horses. *Eq. Vet. J. 1:* 287–289, 1969.
79. Rooney, J. R., Prickett, M. E. and Crowe, M. W. Aortic ring rupture in stallions. *Path. Vet. 4:* 268–274, 1967.
80. Rooney, J. R. Internal hemorrhage related to gestation in the mare. *Cornell Vet. 54:* 11–17, 1964.
81. Rooney, J. R. Volvulus, strangulation, and intussusception in the horse. *Cornell Vet. 55:* 644–653, 1965.
82. Rooney, J. R. Gastric ulceration in foals. *Path. Vet. 1:* 497–503, 1964.
83. Rooney, J. R. The pathology of respiratory diseases of foals. *Proceedings of the First International Congress on Equine Infectious Diseases*, Stresa, 70–75, 1966.
84. Rooney, J. R. Biomechanics of lameness in horses. The Williams & Wilkins Co., Baltimore, 1969.
85. Rooney, J. R. and Jeffcott, L. B. Muscular hypertrophy of the Ileum in a horse. *Vet. Rec. 83:* 215–217, 1968.
86. Rooney, J. R. and Delaney, F. M. Roaring in Horses—A Theoretical Analysis. *Eq. Vet. J.*, in press, 1970.
87. Rooney, J. R. and Franks, W. C. Congenital cardiac anomalies in horses. *Path. Vet. 1:* 454–464, 1964.
88. Ribelin, W. E. Azoturia and the crush syndrome. *J. Amer. Vet. Med. Ass. 69:* 284–288, 1951.
89. Rider, J. R. Diverticula of the small intestine in the horse. *Vet. Rec. 10:* 707–711, 1930.
90. Rider, J. R. Diverticula of the small intestine. *Vet. Rec. 12:* 1202–1206, 1932.
91. Sager, F. C. Personal communications, 1961–1968.
92. Selye, H. *Stress.* Acta, Inc., Montreal, 1950.
93. Schummer, A. Morphologische Untersuchungen uber die Funktionszustände des Ileums. *Tierärztl. Umschau 8:* 244–247, 1953.
94. Soulsby, E. J. L. *Textbook of Veterinary Clinical Parasitology.* F. A. Davis, Philadelphia, 1965.
95. Sparks, J. Personal communication, 1968.
96. Takizawa, N., Murayama, H. and Homma, Y. Five autopsy cases of "Myokardose." *Acta Path. Jap. 8:* 925–935, 1958.
97. Teeter, S. Personal communication, 1969.
98. Theiler, A. Acute liver atrophy and parenchymatous hepatitis in horses. *Rep. Director Vet. Res. S. Afr. 6:* 7–164, 1919.
99. Thurlbeck, W. M. and Lowell, F. C. Heaves in horses. *Amer. Rev. Resp. Dis. 89:* 82–88, 1964.
100. Tudor, D. C. Bibliography of equine infectious anemia. Proceedings of the U.S. Livestock Sanitary Association, 70th Annual Meeting 1966.
101. Van Niekerk, C. H. and Gerneke, W. H. Persistence and parthenogenetic cleavage of tubal ova in the mare. *Onderstepoort. J. Vet. Res. 33:* 195–232, 1966.
102. Vaughan, J. T. and Bartels, J. E. Equine mandibular adamantinoma. *J. Amer. Vet. Med. Ass. 153:* 454–457, 1968.
103. Winqvist, G. Topografisk och etiologisk sammanställning av de fibrinosa och ulcerosa endokarditerna hos en del av våra husdjur. *Skand. Vet-Tidskr. 35:* 575–585, 1945.
104. Zietzschmann, O. and Krölling, O. *Lehrbuch der Entwicklungsgeschichte der Haustiere.* Paul Parey, Berlin, 1955.

APPENDIX 1

Check List for Procedure

1. Place carcass in dorsal recumbency. Cut down all four legs.
2. Skin abdomen and ventral surfaces of throat and neck.
3. Open abdomen—midline.
4. Reflect flanks by cutting along costal arches.
5. Displace cecum and colon to right, descending colon to left, out of abdomen.
6. Displace small intestine out of abdomen to right.
7. Locate duodenocolic ligament. Free ascending duodenum. Transect at caudal flexure.
8. Strip small intestine from mesentery.
9. Transect ileum at ileocecal fold.
10. Remove great mesentery.
11. Transect descending colon at pelvic inlet. Displace to right and strip from mesocolon.
12. Free transverse colon from pancreas by blunt dissection.
13. Isolate and transect cranial mesenteric artery close to aorta.
14. Remove large intestine.
15. Free left and right tails of pancreas by blunt dissection.
16. Isolate and transect branches of celiac artery close to viscus: hepatic, left gastric, splenic.
17. Pull spleen to right. Transect splenorenal and gastrosplenic ligaments and remove spleen.
18. Transect duodenum, esophagus, and remove stomach.
19. Cut right lateral ligament; tear out hepatorenal ligament. Cut left lateral and falciform ligaments. Open caudal vena cava. Remove liver, pancreas, duodenum *en bloc*.
20. Saw and remove block of bone from pelvis.
21. Remove urogenital tract *en toto*.
22. Remove diaphragm.
23. Free sternal attachments of pericardium.
24. Reflect tongue, pharynx, larynx.
25. Transect trachea, esophagus.

26. Remove thoracic viscera.
27. Remove head.
28. Examine forelimb after skinning. Transect flexors and suspensory.
29. Open and examine: digital sheath, navicular area, pastern joint, fetlock, tendons, carpus, elbow, shoulder, bicipital bursa.
30. As forelimb and tibiotarsal joint, stifle, hip.
31. Examine the viscera, in any order, by palpation, inspection, slicing. Determine size, shape, position, color, consistency, cut surface.
32. Collect specimens.
33. Record the findings.

APPENDIX 2

Application of Autopsy Technique to Other Animals

In this appendix I should like to indicate briefly how the autopsy technique described for the horse can be readily and easily adapted to other, and indeed all, species of animals. Since my particular specialty is equine pathology, no attempt will be made to describe the gross pathology of these other species.

One of the major features of the autopsy procedure which has been described is the emphasis on anatomical and functional relationships as the dissection proceeds. When the procedure is applied to other animals, this point is emphasized. The dissection clearly shows the basic similarities and highlights the specific anatomical modifications among species. This is at no time so apparent as during the autopsy of an unfamiliar animal. When the autopsy is complete, the prosector, if he does not know the diagnosis, will at least have a clear picture of the gross anatomy of that animal.

In recent years the concept of a core curriculum with drastic reduction in the number of required hours in the basic medical sciences has been gaining in popularity. It undoubtedly represents a significant and important step forward in medical training. This autopsy procedure, with its emphasis on anatomical dissection, fits this new concept. The student not only learns pathology but is continually reviewing anatomy with every autopsy he performs. With proper guidance, physiology also can be reviewed and pathologic physiology developed within its proper anatomical framework. A discussion of the function of the gall bladder naturally follows as the ducts are traced into the duodenum. The physiological role of the several parts of the digestive tract may be succinctly reviewed as the dissection proceeds systematically.

The ruminant presents the most striking anatomical difference in the complex stomach. Since this is the largest and most voluminous portion of the gastrointestinal tract, it is removed first. The omentum is removed, the duodenum transected just distal to the pylorus, and the entire stomach rolled to the left. Once the omentum is removed (or earlier), the prosector may readily examine the reticular area for the adhesions and inflammation characteristic of traumatic reticulitis. The esophagus is readily located, ligated,* and

* It is wise to always ligate the esophagus of ruminants because of the large quantity of fluid ingesta.

transected. The stomach is rolled farther to the left and the spleen blunt dissected free of its attachments. The weight of the stomach, blunt dissection of the sublumbar attachments of the rumen, and severing the celiac artery will free the stomach complex completely, allowing it to roll out on the floor.

The small intestine is stripped from the mesentery as in the horse, drawing it out on the right side. The descending colon is transected at the pelvic inlet and the colon removed *en bloc*, leaving the pancreas with the liver and duodenum precisely as in the horse. While of little pathological significance in the bovine, the cranial mesenteric artery can be examined or dissected for later examination at this time. If indicated the colon can be unraveled after removal although as a rule it is preferable to open it *in continuum*, so that the site of lesions can be clearly defined.

The right ligament of the ruminant liver is small and ill defined and need not be broken down as in the horse. The falciform ligament is severed, opening the vena cava. The vena cava is split with the hands and examined, and the liver is removed as in the horse. From this point forward the dissection is essentially identical to that of the horse.

Swine, dogs, cats, rats, etc., may be dissected in virtually the same manner as the horse, except that the colon is not displaced. The order of dissection always remains the same, the ruminant being the only exception: small intestine, large intestine, spleen, stomach, liver-pancreas-duodenum, urogenital tract, etc.

Index

Only matters of interpretation are indexed. The dissection procedure is not indexed as the table of contents provides adequate page references.